MYOSITIS

facts, feelings and future hopes

3·99

2 / 14

Editor: Jenny Fenton

Published by *Thoughtful Publications*
First published in Great Britain (2006)

*To Rob with my love and thanks for the years of
love and support*

Dedicated to Ma and Pop

10 July 08

Jn Nna,

Instead of having this
as a reminder when you
leave — Keep it as a
reminder to "Do same work"

Yours

Bernie

Published by Thoughtful Publications
First published in Great Britain July 2003 as 'Living with Myositis'
Second Edition 'Myositis' (revised and expanded) 2006
PO Box 46214 LONDON W5 1YF

Editor: Jennifer Fenton
Assistant Editors: Dr. C. Bernard Colaço, Dr. Robert J. Fenton

Jacket design by Duncan Spilling
Cover Photograph Copyright © Getty Images (UK) Ltd.

Printed and bound in Great Britain by Ideal Printers, Amersham

Typesetting by Angela Wood, Teddington, Middlesex

Sponsored by The Central Middlesex Hospital Rheumatology Trust Fund
With thanks to Dr C. Bernard Colaço

Contents

SECTION FOUR – Understanding the Science

SECTION FIVE – Resources

Foreword

by Dr C. Bernard Colaço BSc (Hons) MBChB FRCP
Consultant Rheumatologist,
Central Middlesex Hospital, Park Royal, London

This second edition is another achievement for Jenny whose remarkable first edition 'Living with Myositis' was a sell out. It has set a standard for the genre of patient focussed publications. The book has been sold to patients and professionals at near cost levels and the modest profit has been directed towards myositis research. What a success! I would have gone for a reprint but Jenny has moved on with a worldwide sister/brotherhood of web friends and she has attracted several new contributors to this wonderful resource, which has been thoroughly refreshed. Jenny's project keeps me personally up to date with myositis, and I wish her luck with this and the inevitable 3rd edition.

Myositis is rare but can be devastating in medical terms, especially in children, but even milder cases can take over the patient's and carers' or family's lives.

Jenny has known me now for perhaps too many years, and I initially offered superficial support to her declaration, 'I will write a book on myositis' (for patients) as she had found researching her own disease quite difficult. This was back in 2000 and resulted in the book '*Living with Myositis*'.

Outcome measures are difficult to quantify and large, properly conducted randomised clinical trials are almost impossible because the condition is so rare.

This possibly fuelled Jenny's enthusiasm and the brief personal monologue which I had originally expected, has flourished into this wonderful project which I believe has bridged the gap between patient information leaflets, and accessing medical literature directly.

Rob and I were enticed into an assistant editorial role, but the dirty work and drive has always been Jenny's, and her cartel of associates from the Central Middlesex Hospital Rheumatology Patient's Self Help Group. Jenny has been their Chairperson for a few years and has also recruited numerous others to the cause of myositis research.

I have been impressed with the quality and sensitivity of the personal views, which I found surprisingly, opened my not inexperienced medical eyes. I commend these essays to all medical students requiring an early insight into the patient's and doctor's role in managing chronic diseases.

The other contributors, including some new ones who are all experts in their field, have willingly given of their time and I am grateful to them. I would also like to thank John McCarthy, Fiona Watt and Mona Manghani who have worked with me in the Central Middlesex Hospital Rheumatology Unit. The service itself, at CMH, has relied heavily upon another close liaison with the laboratory led by Jo Wilson who has been tireless in her service to our patients and has added a new chapter to this edition.

This book will reach a much wider audience than the myositis community as it has gems of insights through all of its now many chapters.

My congratulations again to Jenny, and I am delighted to have been involved and to be able to support this publication from the CMH Rheumatology Trust Fund.

Thanks again Jenny.

Dr Colaço has had an interest in autoimmune mediated diseases since training as an SHO in renal medicine in Bristol. His original publications on ANA negative lupus from the Hammersmith Hospital with Professor Keith Elkon, and pivotal studies on anti-phospholipid antibodies 20 years ago, have led on to significant changes in patient care. He has also studied Rheumatoid families under Professor Ivan Roitt FRS as a research fellow at the Middlesex Hospital, London W1. He heads a lupus/vasculitis clinic in NW London serving a highly susceptible local immigrant population.

Introduction

by Jenny Fenton

Myositis is classified as an autoimmune disorder. However, the cause of myositis is still unknown. The disease is rare, affecting five to ten out of every one million people. Because the disease is rare, people living with myositis often feel isolated, with few to talk to about their condition. Like other rheumatic diseases, myositis is unlikely to resolve on its own. But with proper drug treatment and management, myositis can, in most cases, be brought under control. Without treatment the disease may be severe enough to put the patient's life at risk. The main symptoms of myositis are muscle weakness and extreme fatigue.

Aims

The main purpose for producing this book is to: –

– give support, encouragement and empathy to people with dermatomyositis, polymyositis, inclusion body myositis and juvenile myositis,

– raise awareness of the condition.

– provide information to people living with myositis, their families and carers in order to gain a better understanding of the illness,

– relieve the isolation felt by people living with myositis when they are diagnosed with this severe, rare illness,

– give the medical profession an insight into the feelings and frustrations of patients,

– give hope.

Readership

The chapters in *Myositis* have been written to encompass a wide readership. People with myositis will find *Myositis* an invaluable support, both emotionally and practically.

Family members, friends and carers will gain an understanding into the needs, both emotional and physical, of people with myositis.

The authors, who have contributed to *Myositis*, have considered issues from a variety of different professional and family member perspectives. *Myositis* therefore, provides an important resource for practitioners who are likely to be involved in the care of a person with myositis. This could include doctors, nurses, occupational therapists, physiotherapists and counsellors.

Contents

Myositis contains a range of chapters covering a spectrum of contributions from the personal to the professional. All the contributors however, share a knowledge about the condition either from personal experience – their own, or that of a relative, or from a professional involvement in its treatment.

Any book that contains edited chapters from many contributors will inevitably contain a range of writing styles and content. Because *Myositis* contains this diversity of contributions, some chapters are deeply personal and provide an insight into the impact of myositis and the personality of the author, whilst others are written from a professional perspective, providing clear information and academic references. It is hoped that this will provide something for everyone who encounters myositis and help both the lay person and the medical profession to gain an insight into the condition.

Myositis is divided into five sections.

Section One – The Impact of Myositis starts by giving the reader an overview of myositis covering many different aspects and written in a way that is accessible to all. It has been written by Dr Geraldine Cambridge and Dr Rob Fenton. After the initial overview it leads naturally into the 'case studies' beginning with the editor's own story and then into stories and updates from people with dermatomyositis

(DM), polymyositis (PM), inclusion body myositis (IBM) and juvenile myositis (JDM). The stories written by people with JDM are particularly moving. Many of their parents have also written about how it was for them to have a young child with JDM. A chapter on 'remission' with several case studies and an introduction by Richard Gay, who himself has JDM/DM, completes Section One.

Section Two – Living with Myositis helps the patient to cope with the emotional side of having a chronic illness. The editor, Jenny Fenton, has written '*Is this Myositis*' which focuses on the strange often worrying symptoms that people sometimes experience. It is often comforting to know that you are not alone. '*Emotions, Empathy and Encouragement*' has been compiled by Jenny but has been written by people with myositis. Readers who have myositis will identify with the emotions. Angela Hunter has written the next chapter on coping with stress, the impact of myositis on relationships and coping with myositis during the holidays. Angela coordinates a free monthly Myositis Support Group, offered as a community service by the Hospital for Special Surgery, New York, USA. Lisa Copen, who is the founder and director of 'Rest Ministries' in the USA, writes about how hard it can be living with an 'invisible' illness. Lisa lives with rheumatoid arthritis and fibromyalgia and is the author of '*When Chronic Illness Enters Your Life Bible Study*'. A clear, concise explanation of counselling is described in '*Counselling and Myositis*' by Dr William West.

Section Three – Therapies concentrates on treatment, ranging from conventional medicine to nutrition. Dr Rob Fenton, who has worked in the pharmaceutical industry for over thirty years, gives us an overview of current medical treatment. In '*Nutrition*', Audrey Howe gives us invaluable advice on what to eat for optimum health (within the confines of having an autoimmune illness). She answers many of the questions we ask including how to avoid osteoporosis and how to keep our blood sugar levels steady, both of which can be problems as a result of taking steroids. Julie Mallen, who trained as an occupational therapist since having had myositis herself, gives us a detailed insight into how occupational therapy can help in some cases. Section Three concludes with Dr Selwyn Richards telling us about different types of exercise, which is advisable and which is not so advisable, how to motivate yourself and how to stick to an exercise programme. Helene Alexandersson, a physiotherapist from the Karolinska Institute in Sweden has devised, after much research, an exercise programme for people with myositis. Illustrations accompany the programme.

Section Four – Understanding the Science is a heavier read and begins with a chapter on genetics. Dr Hector Chinoy, Professor William Ollier and Dr Robert Cooper give an introduction to the possible genetic links of myositis, even though the cause of idiopathic inflammatory myopathies is still unknown. In the following chapter Yannoulla (Jo) Wilson, who is head of immunology at a west London hospital, takes us through the problems met when diagnosing autoimmune disease and subsequent laboratory testing. Susan Maillard, who is a physiotherapist, and Dr Lucy Wedderburn, who is reader and consultant in paediatric rheumatology give an overview of myositis in children. An informative account of inclusion body myositis is given by Dr John McCarthy. The possible complication of lung disease has been addressed by Dr Mona Manghani and Dr Fiona Watt. Theresa Curry, who works for The Myositis Association of America, has kindly given us her report on '*Dysphagia*'.

Section Five – Resources is equally as important as the other sections and begins with a page compiled by Janet Horton on how to claim disability allowance. Janelle Jones, herself a JDM patient, gives us valuable information on makeup to camouflage the DM rash. Plus at the end of this section there is a resource section and glossary which explains all those difficult medical terms.

As can be seen from the description of the contents, *Myositis* is intended to be used by people with myositis, health care professionals, carers and friends. It is the intention of the editor to give people practical advice, support and empathy but most of all hope.

SECTION ONE

The Impact of Myositis

1

What is Myositis?
– an introduction

by Geraldine Cambridge B.Sc. (Hons), Ph.D.
Honorary Lecturer (Rheumatology/Immunology)
Department of Medicine, University College London, UK

and Rob Fenton BSc (Hons), PhD

Myositis means inflammation of the muscles. 'Poly' means many, 'myo' means muscle, 'itis' means inflammation and 'derma' means skin.

The inflammatory myopathies (myositis diseases) affect individuals differently and are probably caused by several different factors. Few cases are identical or follow the same pattern. They are thought to be immune mediated. In healthy people, the immune system attacks bacteria and viruses that cause disease. In people with an autoimmune disease, there is a defect in the immune system that causes it to turn against the body's own tissues or 'self'. Some doctors feel that myositis may be caused by a virus or certain drugs, plus a possible genetic predisposition to develop an autoimmune disease, but the definitive reason for acquiring this disease is not known. In rare instances, IBM has been seen in families ("familial" IBM). To date, it isn't known whether this disease is directly inherited (a defective gene) or whether the susceptibility to acquiring the disease through external factors, is inherited. Hereditary inclusion body myopathy (h-IBM), is however a proven genetic disease. This disease, like IBM, is characterised by muscle weakness and the presence of inclusion bodies. However, in this disease, there is no associated muscle inflammation as seen in IBM.

Some people may develop myositis over months or even years before it is noticed and as these diseases are relatively rare, diagnosis can take a long time. However, the majority will find that within weeks they have developed muscle weakness. Sometimes pain and tenderness accompany this. As a result, the patient usually experiences difficulty in walking, lifting arms, or getting up out of a chair. There may also be difficulty in swallowing and the voice may become husky. In children particularly, a general feeling of misery and depression is very noticeable and can be an indication of the disease before any sign of muscle weakness.

Polymyositis and dermatomyositis are related illnesses affecting muscle and connective tissues of the body. Inclusion body myositis is usually progressive and more difficult to treat. Children can develop polymyositis (known as Juvenile Polymyositis or JPM) or dermatomyositis (Juvenile Dermatomyositis or JDM); however, dermatomyositis is the more common (see below). Inclusion body myositis is unknown in children.

Polymyositis

Polymyositis (PM) is usually a disease of adults with the average age of onset from 50-60 years. The development of the condition is often slow with weakness of the neck, upper arm and leg muscles being most common. In nearly half of patients, other tissues such as the joints, heart and lungs can be involved. Myositis can also occur as part of an overlap with other so-called 'connective tissue diseases' such as lupus and also with autoimmune diseases affecting other tissues such as the thyroid, salivary glands (Sjogrens syndrome), the intestine (e.g. Coeliac disease, Crohn's disease) and the joints (Rheumatoid arthritis).

Dermatomyositis

The pattern of muscle weakness in Dermatomyositis (DM) is similar to that in PM but onset can be more sudden and dramatic. The condition can also occur in children; PM being rare in children (DM:PM 25:1). Difficulty in swallowing (dysphagia) is more common in DM. The accompanying skin rash is usually very distinctive and virtually diagnostic of DM. It consists of a red, scaly rash of the face (particularly over the eyelids), neck, back and upper arms with marked red, often raised patches over the joints.

Inclusion body myositis

IBM is a slowly progressive muscle disease often seen in the over fifty's, but in very rare instances has been diagnosed in younger persons. Like PM and DM, IBM is an inflammatory condition of the muscles. However, unlike DM and PM, muscle weakness progresses slowly, with a painless weakening of a specific limb or limbs, such as the muscles of the thighs (quadriceps), lower legs, arms, wrists and fingers. In a number of patients (20-40%), the muscles of the oesophagus can also be affected, causing difficulty in swallowing (dysphagia). The symptoms of this disease usually first appear in those over the age of 50, but rarely can occur in younger persons. IBM appears to be more common in males than in females. Unlike PM and DM, IBM appears to be a lot more resistant to conventional therapies. However, in some patients, prednisolone has shown benefit, and more recently there have been reports of some patients showing improvement with intravenous immunoglobulin (IVIG).

Because of the similarities in presentation, IBM is often diagnosed as either PM or DM. However, a definitive diagnosis can be made by taking muscle biopsies. These biopsies, when viewed microscopically, are characterised by the presence of intracellular amyloid protein deposits, or 'inclusion bodies'.

Juvenile Dermatomyositis

In juvenile dermatomyositis, the skin symptoms are much more likely to appear before muscle symptoms; the reverse being true for the adult form of this disease. The clinical picture in children also often seems to reflect a more widespread disease affecting small blood vessels in tissues other than skin and muscle, especially those of the digestive system. In addition, deposits of calcium compounds in muscle and skin are often a major problem in children with DM. Unlike adult dermatomyositis, there appears to be no association in children with DM, with an increased rate of cancers.

Juvenile polymyositis has a clinical picture similar to that of adult polymyositis, and so is not discussed here further. (See separate chapter 'Myositis in Children').

Frequently asked questions

Q. *How did I get this illness?*
A. Some doctors feel that myositis may be caused by a virus or certain drugs, plus a possible genetic predisposition to develop an autoimmune disease, but the definitive reason for acquiring this disease is not known.

Q. *Can I pass the disease on to my family and friends?*
A. No, the disease cannot be passed on to other people. It is a disorder of the body, rather than being an infectious disease.

Q. *Is my illness life threatening?*
A. Without treatment DM/PM has an increased mortality rate, though IBM doesn't. With the correct treatment the illness should be managed. It should also be noted that immunosuppresive therapies can lead to a greater susceptibility to opportunistic infections.

Q. *I've heard that there is an increased risk of cancer in patients with myositis, is this true?*
A. There is an increased rate of cancer in adults with DM, though this isn't apparent in adults with PM or IBM. Whether cancers are the result of the onset of DM or vice versa, is not known. Some physicians still find this association over emphasised as the cancer may have been diagnosed years before or after the onset of DM.

Q. *I've heard I should keep out of bright sunlight, is this true?*
A. Yes this is true for DM/PM and JDM/JPM patients, as it can cause a 'flare'.

Q. *Are there any effective treatments?*
A. There are now a number of treatments available, and in the majority of patients these can be very effective in reducing the severity of the disease. Most treatments act by reducing the inflammatory process by inhibiting the immune system. Patients with DM, PM, JDM/JPM appear to benefit the most, with IBM patients generally being unresponsive (see IBM chapter).

Q. *Do the treatments have any side effects?*
A. All effective treatments have side effects. The most commonly used 'first-line' treatments are steroids (e.g. prednisone/prednisolone). Steroids are associated with a number of side effects including weight gain (increased appetite), 'moon-face', hair thinning, hair loss, increased facial hair (in women), skin thinning, poor sleep patterns and perhaps most importantly bone loss (osteoporosis). Bone (Dexa) scans are recommended as soon as steroid therapy commences to establish a base line bone density followed by further bone scans to establish the presence of bone loss (osteopaenia) and subsequent osteoporosis. Osteopaenia and subsequent osteoporosis can be slowed down/inhibited by treatment with drugs that aid the re-absorption of calcium (e.g. Fosamax (alendronate) and Didronel PMO (etidronate disodium).

All of the side effects of steroid therapy are most apparent during the initial phase of treatment when doses are high. As the doses are reduced, these effects also reduce.

Methotrexate may also be responsible for a persistent cough. However, in some patients persistent cough can be a complication of the disease itself (interstitial lung disease).

Q. *Will I get better?*
A. Patients treated early and aggressively benefit the most, with a high proportion of patients achieving partial or complete remission. However, as treatment protocols are reduced (e.g. lowering the dose), the disease may re-appear (flare) and the treatment may need to be stepped up again.

Q. *How long will I need treatment?*
A. Treatment is likely to be long term. Most patients require treatment for a minimum of two years; any less and the disease is more likely to re-occur (flare). In some patients, treatment can be for life. In patients treated with steroids, high doses may initially be given (60mg+), this dose slowly tapering down over the next few months/years.

Q. *Will I start to feel better as soon as I start treatment?*
A. Many patients report feeling an immediate benefit when treatment starts with high dose steroid; however, some patients

feel a lot worse for the first few weeks of treatment. The reasons for this are unclear and again it seems to be down to the fact that we all react differently.

Q. *If I start to feel better can I stop treatment?*
A. The answer is no. There is no quick fix to these diseases. Stopping treatment prematurely will usually result in a flare, and you will have to start all over again. Patients on steroids must never stop taking the treatment suddenly, as this can be very dangerous. Steroids **must always** be reduced slowly.

Q. *I've heard it can be difficult getting off steroids, is this true?*
A. Most patients find it relatively easy to taper their dose down from 60mg to 10mg, but it gets increasingly more difficult to taper from 10mg to zero. In some patients, getting below 5mg may take time as your adrenal glands start to kick in again. Long-term steroid treatment can also lead to steroid dependence in a proportion of patients whose adrenal glands have become sluggish. In these patients a maintenance dose of steroids may be necessary for life.

Q. *What if I get pregnant?*
A. First of all the myositis condition shouldn't affect your baby. However, some mothers do experience the symptoms of myositis getting worse during pregnancy. Secondly, the medicines you take will get into baby's bloodstream, so it is very important to request pre-conceptual counselling from your obstetrician and you must tell your consultant as soon as you get pregnant. Steroids are safe to take during pregnancy, though they have been linked with an increased incidence of premature babies. However, it is essential that some medicines are avoided. These include methotrexate, cyclophosphamide and possibly hydroxychloroquine. It is also important to note that medicines will also get through to mother's milk. Although the levels of medicines passed on to baby through breast-feeding tend to be much lower than that passed on during pregnancy, it is still important to discuss this with your consultant or pediatrician.

Q. *Why do I need regular blood tests?*
A. Blood samples can give all sorts of information as to a) how the disease is progressing/regressing and b) whether or not the

treatments are causing any toxic effects. The most useful predictor of disease regression in some patients, is that of the creatine kinase (CK or CPK). This enzyme is a muscle specific indicator of inflammation. 'Normal' levels vary between 25 and 200u/l (though athletes may have higher levels during periods of exercise). Patients first diagnosed with myositis may have levels in the thousands (or even tens of thousands). In addition, the presence of 'self' or autoimmune antibodies (e.g. anti-nuclear antibody (ANA), anti dsDNA antibody, anti-mitochondrial antibody etc.) give a good diagnosis of disease, and can also be an indicator of disease regression. Patients on steroids need to keep an eye on potassium levels, as low levels of potassium in the bloodstream will lead to weakness and other side effects such as heart irregularities. The levels can by regulated by taking potassium supplements, but only under your doctor's guidance (e.g. SANDO K, SLOW K).

Q. *I get tingling in my scalp and other parts of my body. Is this related to my illness?*
A. This phenomenon is often described by myositis patients. Whether it is disease related, or treatment related isn't known.

Answers compiled by:
Rob Fenton BSc (Hons), PhD

2

What is Myositis?
– history, what happens and hope

by Geraldine Cambridge B.Sc. (Hons), Ph.D.
Honorary Lecturer (Rheumatology/Immunology)
Department of Medicine, University College London

The history of myositis

In 1863 a young German physician named Erlich Wagner described a patient with an 'acute progressive generalised muscle affection' associated with a pronounced skin rash. Over 20 years later, again in Germany, an account of a similar case was reported, although without skin involvement. In the same year, Wagner described a further case of what he called 'polymyositis', with symptoms similar to the earlier reported case. The term 'dermatomyositis' was first used in 1887 because of the florid skin rash accompanying the muscle weakness in the condition. In 1891, Unverrich, another physician, noticed that the upper or 'proximal' limbs were most affected and made the observation that spontaneous recovery could also occur. The occasional involvement of other muscle tissues, for example in the eye and the heart, was first reported in 1899 and 1903. Most of these early observations reported the disease as being acute in onset and rapidly progressive but others described a form of the disease with a course which progressed more slowly.

Most of the early descriptions of this clinical condition were from Germany. In the first cases in the UK (Gowers 1899) the term 'polymyositis' was used to describe the disease despite the fact that both patients had obvious skin involvement. This seemed to emphasise the clinical similarity of the muscle symptoms in patients either with or without skin disease and for many years, the terms polymyositis and dermatomyositis were used interchangeably. In the last 50 years, the classifications most used by clinicians in the field have recognized that skin involvement may be a major component of the disease and when present, the term 'dermatomyositis' should be used. If it is completely absent, the term 'polymyositis' is the preferred term. However, even today, there may still be confusion as to which category to use when the rash is atypical or transient in nature.

Early modern research and the development of standard diagnostic criteria were largely based at the Mayo Clinic and University of California in the US and in Newcastle in the UK.

The two adult forms of myositis have therefore been described for nearly 150 years and the disease in children has also been recognised for many years.

As long ago as 1966 (Banker and Victor) argued the case for a distinction between the diseases which occurred in adults and children. The major difference cited was that in the childhood form of the disease, DM was 25 times more common than PM compared with a 2:1 ratio of PM:DM in adults. It was also suggested that in the dermatomyositis of childhood, the skin symptoms were much more likely to appear before muscle symptoms. The clinical picture in children also often seems to reflect a more widespread disease affecting small blood vessels in tissues other than skin and muscle, especially those of the digestive system. In addition, deposits of calcium compounds in muscle and skin are often a major problem in children with DM. However, many adult patients with DM can also have what appears to be a more systemic type of condition, with joint, heart and lung involvement. Some patients (up to 40%) with PM can also have the disease affecting tissues other than muscle. This usually takes the form of another connective tissue disorder such as lupus (in which almost any other tissue can be involved) or Sjogren's syndrome (dry eyes and mouth) or a myositis with severe lung involvement (so-called 'Jo-1 antibody' associated muscle/lung disease). In adults with DM (not children) there is some association of the condition with a wide range of cancers namely breast and ovarian in women and lung and colon in males. Some clinicians still find this association to be over emphasised as the tumour may have been diagnosed years before or after the onset of DM.

* NOTE: I have not put in a separate section on PM and DM in children as the general descriptions of the tests and clinical features in adults with DM do closely resemble the condition in children. However, I have tried to include the special problems and complications of myositis in children throughout the text – see separate chapter. *Inclusion body myositis is discussed in a separate chapter.*

What happens when you develop myositis?

Despite most early descriptions in which the disease was noted to be 'acute' or sudden in onset, PM is now more commonly regarded as becoming evident in the patient over weeks, months or even years. The proximal (upper) muscles are usually the first affected so the initial symptoms may be a noticeable difficulty in climbing stairs or rising from a chair. Muscle pain and tenderness are symptoms in only some patients (<50%). Occasionally, an acute, painful but very limited form of the disease has been described in which only a single or a limited number of muscles is affected. The often distressing symptom of difficulty in swallowing (*dysphagia*) is due to involvement of the muscles of the pharynx (throat) – *see separate chapter*. Other related features such as Raynaud's phenomenon (fingers turning blue-white in the cold) and evidence of joint or lung involvement can occur in a minority of PM patients. When the 'typical' skin rash accompanies the muscle symptoms, the term dermatomyositis is used. The rash most frequently consists of a purplish discoloration of the eyelids, sometimes accompanied by swelling around the eyes, and scaly, red changes in the skin of the hands and face which can extend over the large joints and whole upper body. Unusual, localised and/or transient skin rashes can complicate classification of patients as belonging to either group.

The tiredness, lack of appetite and sometimes clinical depression suffered by many PM and DM patients are often a major, and often under-treated part of the disease course. In children, general misery, associated with not wanting to join in games, is often the first symptom.

Diagnosis of myositis

A number of different underlying causes can result in the symptoms of myositis. For example chronic (continuous) infection of the muscle with bacteria, parasites or virus, certain poisons or toxins, genetically determined conditions such as the muscular dystrophies and inclusion body myositis can also give a biopsy picture similar to that seen in the so-called immune mediated diseases of PM and DM. Clinicians have therefore compiled guidelines for the diagnosis of these conditions.

The most commonly used of these for the diagnosis of inflammatory muscle disease, which includes PM and DM was published by Bohan and Peter in 1975. This rests on five major criteria. There is still however, considerable controversy about how rigorously these criteria must be met for the diagnosis to be made in individual cases.

1 Progressive muscle weakness

Affected muscles may include the upper muscles of the arms and legs, muscles of the neck, abdomen and those supporting the spine, the respiratory muscles and those involved with swallowing.

2 Elevation of blood levels of enzymes associated with muscle damage

These include most notably creatine kinase (CK or CPK), aldolase, lactate dehydrogenase, aspartate aminotransferase, and alanine aminotransferase. All except CK however, can be made by the liver in response to inflammation so are not really 'muscle specific'.

3 Muscle biopsy changes

Normal muscle tissue, taken from the leg or arm, when cut crosswise and viewed under the microscope, looks like a regular area of roundish paving stones. Each paving stone represents one muscle cell or fibre. The nuclei of mature muscle cells (which unlike most other cells have more than one nucleus) lie at the rim. The muscle cells lie in groups called 'fascicles' bounded by thicker bands of loose connective tissue in which larger blood vessels lie. In myositis, the muscle cells appear much more variable in shape and size, with lots of 'small' cells with central nuclei. The spaces between the cells can be greatly increased and filled with lots of connective or scar tissue (also called fibrosis), muscle cells trying to undergo repair and abundant so-called chronic inflammatory cells (macrophages and lymphocytes) derived from the blood. Some of these cells, the macrophages (literally 'big eaters'), can be seen engulfing muscle cells and producing inflammatory products called cytokines which can further drive the inflammatory response. Smaller round cells called lymphocytes however, usually can also make up a large proportion of the invading blood cells. (A more detailed analysis of 'what is going on' in affected tissue will be presented later in the chapter under Immunology).

4 Electromyographic changes

This investigation consists of measuring the electrical activity in the muscle with a very fine needle. The pattern of the electrical signal can help distinguish between whether the weakness is due to a problem with the muscle or is more likely to be a problem with the nervous system.

5 Skin rash

As already described, the rash most typically takes the form of dry, scaly patches particularly over the hands and around the eyes. However, the rash can extend over most of the body or form discreet, often fleeting patches. Also associated with the skin rash are problems with the finger and often toe-nail beds which are often very brittle and scaly, resulting too in split, broken nails.

Current Measures of disease activity: uses and pitfalls

Once the diagnosis of either PM or DM is made, the difficult process of monitoring disease activity begins. There is considerable variation from patient to patient even within the parameters used for diagnosis, let alone when trying to measure the activity of the disease. The most commonly used measures of disease activity are muscle strength tests, serum levels of CK and other enzymes and repeat muscle biopsies.

• *Muscle biopsy*

The muscle biopsy at diagnosis may be normal in up to 30% of cases, even when weakness is severe. This is probably because of the very patchy nature of the inflammation. Badly affected muscle fibres can be surrounded by perfectly normal ones. As an aid to finding the best place to biopsy, a relatively new technique called MRI (magnetic resonance imaging) is sometimes used in specialist centres. This technique detects inflammation by measuring the relative proportion of water in different tissues. The more inflammation, the more the tissue is likely to be damaged and therefore 'leaky'. Repeat muscle biopsies are therefore not as useful as would be expected unless 'guided' to the most affected tissue by MRI or other inflammation detecting techniques.

They are however useful in order the check that the diagnosis is correct, particularly in cases where the patient has not responded to conventional treatment, for example in inclusion body myositis. Repeat muscle biopsies can be distressing to some patients (and to researchers – personal experience – GC!) and are now only usually done under general anaesthetic in children. Repeat muscle biopsies can therefore potentially give the clinician useful information about whether the disease is present, whether it is active or not and importantly, what the level of fibrosis or scarring is in the muscle. This gives an indication of the long-term prospect of recovery of muscle strength. However, new imaging techniques, such as MRI, will hopefully soon greatly reduce the incidence of repeat muscle biopsies.

• *Measurement of muscle specific markers in blood:*
Of the muscle specific substances released into the bloodstream, creatine kinase (CK) is the most often measured. Again, this can be within 'normal' limits in up to 20% of patients (normal ranges vary considerably between different laboratories and therefore comparisons between serial samples are only valid if tested in the same laboratory). The CK is thought to reflect a balance between muscle breakdown and the ability of the body's scavenging system to get rid of the debris. This will again, vary enormously from patient to patient depending on the area of muscle affected, the 'type' of muscle damage, the disposal capacity of the patient's clean-up (phagocytic) system, stabilisation of muscle membranes by treatment with steroids or other drugs, amongst as yet unknown other factors. Some patients may be extremely weak and have a CK in the low hundreds for example, whilst another may have a CK in the thousands and have nearly normal strength. The overall result is that the CK does not always correlate with disease activity in all patients but does give an indication of disease progression/control in an INDIVIDUAL patient. Measurement of another muscle specific protein called myoglobin, is also used as a soluble measure of muscle damage in some centres.

• *More general laboratory tests*
Serological measures of the overall 'pro-inflammatory' status of the patient can also be used for serial studies of a patient's disease activity. For example, the CRP (C–reactive protein produced by the liver) level

reflects the production of pro-inflammatory substances by the immune cells in the body. ESR is a simple laboratory test of the rate of red cell settling by gravity in a column of blood. Inflammation alters a variety of proteins and glycoproteins in blood which changes the viscosity (stickiness) and allows red cells to settle more rapidly i.e. a raised ESR above the normal range can be monitored for response to therapy, which would hopefully bring it back to the normal range.

• *Immunological tests*
PM and DM are included in a group of conditions known collectively as the autoimmune rheumatic diseases (ARD) in which autoimmune or anti-self responses are thought to underlie the disease process. The hallmark of autoimmune diseases is the presence of antibodies which recognise normal components of cells and/or tissues – the so-called autoantibodies.

A number of autoantibodies have been associated with myositis (*myositis associated autoantibodies*). These autoantibodies have names such as anti-Ro, La, Sm and PM/Scl 75 and are commonly found in conditions such as Sjogrens syndrome, lupus and scleroderma. The 'name' of an antibody usually describes the origin of the antibody e.g. the antibody called Sm was first described in the serum from a patient called Smith! Others are named with the initials of the sub-cellular particle with which they react e.g. anti-SRP denotes antibodies to signal recognition protein.

Others have been shown to be present ONLY in patients with myositis (*myositis specific autoantibodies*) and include such autoantibodies as anti-Jo-1, other anti-synthetase antibodies, anti-Mi and anti-SRP. More than half of patients with myositis have autoantibodies of one or other specificity. Autoantibodies can help diagnosis and to identify disease subsets with distinctive patterns of clinical manifestations, genetics, responses to therapy and prognosis. For example, 75% of PM patients with lung involvement have autoantibodies of the Jo-1 specificity whereas only 20% of patients without lung disease have anti-Jo-1. Children with DM virtually never have anti-Jo-I antibodies and other recognised myositis specific autoantibodies are also rarely found. Patients with anti-SRP tend to have less aggressive disease. As a measure of disease activity, most of these autoantibodies have only limited use, with serial measurements overall being unhelpful. This may be because of a number of complex factors, including the fact that the sub-population of autoantibodies involved in the disease process may be very small, different factors or autoantibodies may be important at different phases of the disease process and the effect of therapy on antibody producing cells. However, because myositis-specific autoantibodies are often associated with distinct clinical profiles, classification according to autoantibody profiles in the future could help to define the cause of different patterns of disease and suggest more appropriate treatments.

Myositis: the damaging process (Pathogenesis)

• **How does the immune system go wrong?**

Patients with autoimmune diseases do not have a general 'breakdown' in their immune system. Conditions such as Rheumatoid arthritis, vasculitis, lupus, coeliac disease, thyroid disease are strongly associated with the presence of only particular autoantibodies in their blood. The type of autoantibodies present are often specific for that condition. In order to understand the nature of autoimmunity it may be helpful to have a brief outline of the normal functioning of the immune system.

• **How the immune system works**

The spectrum of antibodies present in the blood are primarily the result of an encounter between the immune system of the individual and bacteria, viruses, other micro-organisms and environmental factors such as components of food, certain drugs, insect bites etc. The role of antibodies in infections is to lock onto micro–organisms and neutralise them through their ability to attract and attach to inflammatory cells which can then ingest and destroy the invaders. Antibodies can also recognise virus-specific markers on the surface of infected cells (viruses can only live INSIDE living cells) and again by attracting killer lymphocytes, focus the anti-viral attack only on infected cells. The immune system is an extremely complex system of cells and of soluble factors produced by these cells ('cytokines') designed to distinguish non-self from self in order to protect us from microbes in general. The learning process involved in the education of immune cells mostly takes place during prenatal development but does also continue throughout life. The cornerstone of this ability to distinguish self from non-self is the way that bits of bugs or other molecular species (generally called antigens) are 'presented' to the immune cells or lymphocytes. This 'presentation' of antigens is most commonly via other cells called macrophages and dendritic cells which are adept at processing and concentrating possible antigens and in communicating with large numbers of lymphocytes in lymph nodes and the spleen. If the antigen is presented in association with certain pro–inflammatory markers on the presenting cell and in the presence of other 'danger' signals, an immune response is mounted.

• **T–cells and B–cells**
The immune cells or lymphocytes are comprised of 2 basic types – the T (for thymus–derived) and B (bursa or bone marrow derived) lymphocytes. The T lymphocytes or T-cells are regarded by some as the clever clogs and the B cells as the slaves of the T cells. Recently however, the potentially subversive tactics of the B cell have begun to be recognised. Following stimulation by a particular antigen, the T cells and B cells undergo a series of divisions resulting in a large number of now activated cells recognising the same antigen (so–called 'clonal expansion'). These cells are now ready to attack the invader, although some become memory cells which go to hide in the lymph nodes ready for the next encounter with the same stimulus. This accounts for what is called 'specific immunological memory' in that the next time that particular bug is encountered, there are already a number of committed, specific, T or B cells ready to mount a rapid response. This forms the basis of immunisation in that injection with a killed or inactivated bug (e.g. flu virus) results in the expansion of a number of 'flu-specific' T and B cells which will be ready to prevent infection with any related flu virus.

T cells can be divided into two basic types– CD4 or CD8 positive T cells. The CD4 +ve T cells can basically do two things following priming to a particular antigen a) they can make cytokines capable of activating other potentially inflammatory cells and also of damaging tissue cells and b) they provide the necessary signals for the B cells to turn into antibody-producing 'plasma' cells. The CD8 +ve T cells can kill target cells on contact. Each clone of T cells will be specific for the antigen which stimulated its expansion. Following antigen stimulation and clonal expansion, B cells change into large plasma cells which are basically antibody producing factories. These plasma cell can live and produce antibody for a few weeks to years, possibly depending on the type of stimulus initially received. Of the lymphocytes in the circulation, only 5% are of the B type–the remainder being T lymphocytes.

• **Why is myositis an autoimmune disease?**
Inclusion of PM and DM within the group of autoimmune rheumatic diseases has resulted from the finding of autoantibodies in the blood of most patients, the presence of large numbers of lymphocytes in affected tissues and at least a partial response to treatment with drugs known to target the immune system. However, as yet the precise molecular targets for autoimmune attack in myositis and even the way in which tissue damage is caused is not fully understood.

• **A possible role for autoantibodies**
Circumstantial evidence suggests a damaging role for autoantibodies in a number of autoimmune diseases. For example, in myasthenia gravis, a condition where a disruption in nerve-muscle signalling causes muscle weakness, autoantibodies can be detected which bind to the nerve/muscle junction. In some diseases, fluctuations of autoantibody levels in blood correlates with disease activity. They can also be seen deposited in inflammatory sites or bound to the surface of specific target tissues. However, the self-antigens recognised by the serum autoantibodies found in myositis (see above) and other autoimmune rheumatic diseases such as lupus, are usually only found inside cells, and are therefore usually not available to be bound by the autoantibodies in the circulation. However, in patients with DM, but not PM, there is some evidence that antibodies and other serum proteins able to bind antibodies (collectively called complement proteins) are deposited in the small blood vessels of skin and muscle. It has however recently been shown that many of the antigens usually found inside cells can be expressed on cells undergoing a controlled form of cell death called 'apoptosis'. Apoptosis of a cell can be induced following a death signal from a specific CD8+ve T cell. It may be that this process supplies intracellular antigens to the immune system.

The way in which these autoantibodies may contribute to the expression of myositis is not known but likely to be extremely complex. It is certainly not a simple case of the antibodies binding to the surface of muscle or skin cells and causing damage. Even when antibodies are present in affected tissues of patients, they are found deposited in the blood vessels of the muscle or skin, not on the tissue cells themselves. In addition, anti-muscle or skin cell autoantibodies have not been detected in the blood of patients.

• **What are the lymphocytes doing in myositis?**

As discussed in the section on diagnosis, the cells in the inflammatory infiltrate in muscle biopsies from myositis patients consists of macrophages and lymphocytes. The role of macrophages in both conditions is thought to be related to their function in engulfing and removing debris from damaged tissues. Macrophages and also T cells, are also the source of a number of powerful substances called 'cytokines'. These cytokines have the potential to kill or damage tissue cells (e.g. 'tumour necrosis factor alpha-TNFα), protect tissue cells from virus attack (interferon), help drive antibody production (interleukin 4), or, in the case of interleukin 1 produced mainly by macrophages, help T cells to initiate an immune response. In biopsies from PM and DM patients, inflammatory infiltrates are usually patchy in distribution and are often associated with areas of scarring or fibrosis. There have been several studies of the cytokines present in muscle and in blood from patients but no clear association with any particular cytokine (s) has yet been found. There are reportedly differences in the composition and distribution of the infiltrate between biopsies from DM and PM patients. In DM particularly, in biopsies from children with the disease, the inflammatory cells are usually grouped around small intramuscular blood vessels which often show evidence of activation or damage. This can be associated with evidence of antibody deposits in the vessels. Both types of T cells are usually present. In addition, B lymphocytes are often seen near blood vessels in muscle tissue from patients with DM. B lymphocyte survival outside the lymphoid tissues is unusual and depends on the presence of a number of factors and could provide an interesting avenue for investigation. In the skin, obvious inflammation is extremely rare. Small blood vessels often show signs of damage and they are often markedly reduced in number. The overall impression given by the type of damage seen in DM is of a pathogenic process originating from the circulation and focussed on and around the blood vessels.

The infiltrates in biopsies from patients with PM are again variable in intensity and distribution. The predominant T cell type is CD8+ve. These can be seen close to regenerating muscle fibres and also invading apparently normal muscle fibres with long foot–like processes. The products of their cell killing apparatus (hole punching molecules called 'perforins') can occasionally also be seen on muscle cells. When the CD8+ve cells from muscle biopsies are examined in detail, they often show evidence of clonality i.e. they were probably derived and expanded from a restricted population of ancestor CD8+ve T cells. Although this would appear to suggest that the invading CD8+ve T cells were indeed directed against some particular muscle antigen, CD8+ve T cells from muscle biopsies from patients with muscular dystrophy and other non-autoimmune muscle diseases also show restricted clonality. This association of CD8+ve cells with muscle is also of interest because of a possible role for CD8+ve cells in muscle regeneration. The environment in NORMAL muscle tissue is particularly 'friendly' for CD8+ve T cells to move through and they can often be seen in muscle biopsies from normal individuals, especially following exercise induced damage. Many cytokines and other factors from CD8+ve T cells, muscle fibers themselves, and blood vessels have been shown to influence muscle cell regeneration (regrowth) in culture. The association between normal muscle regeneration and the immune system has only recently regained some attention and may provide useful clues for what might be happening in a pathogenic situation such as in PM.

(Pathogenesis) Conclusions

Given the range of findings in the blood of different patients with myositis (e.g. different autoantibodies, levels of muscle enzymes), together with the lack of much consistency in biopsy findings between different patients (e.g. degree and type of inflammation, degree of muscle cell damage), my personal view is that conventional ways of looking at the pathogenesis of myositis are not likely to be productive. It is possible however that the inconsistencies reflect differences in the time point at which we see individual patients. For example, there may be an 'early' phase lasting for varying times between patients where muscle is damaged by an insult such as an infection, some kind of toxin or insect bite (very hypothetical) or as the result of some other condition or disease in the patient, which could perhaps reversibly affect muscle tissue. This could be followed by another phase which would determine the long term functional effects on muscle which are dependent on the extent of replacement of muscle tissue by connective tissue and fat. This may relate to how extensive the damage had been to the muscles, the ability to repair the damage, whether and what type of autoantibodies had been produced, and the composition and degree of inflammation. Whether and which treatment to give patients with myositis would therefore be dependent on the phase of the disease in individual patients.

SUMMARY

Polymyositis (PM) and dermatomyositis (DM) are conditions in which muscle and the skin are targets of what is thought to be an autoimmune attack. The result of this inflammatory attack on these tissues is scarring or fibrosis which results in muscle weakness in both PM and DM and the florid skin rash of DM. Both PM and DM are associated with particular autoantibodies (anti-self antibodies) in the circulation. The way in which autoantibodies contribute to the disease process is not known but indirect evidence of their involvement, particularly in DM, can be found in antibody-containing deposits in blood vessels in skin and muscle tissue from affected patients. A lymphocyte-mediated attack on muscle cells is also thought to be important in the pathogenesis of myositis.

Despite the wide variety of available therapeutic options, up to 25% of patients with myositis remain only partly responsive to therapy either because the treatment itself fails or the patient experiences unacceptable side effects. Treatment of patients at present is with drugs aimed at intervening in the disease process in a general way. For example, corticosteroids decrease inflammation and stop potentially damaging lymphocytes from getting out of the circulation, immunosuppressives (aza-thioprine, cyclophosphamide, cyclosporine, methotrexate) reduce the activity and proliferation of immune cells (lymphocytes). Intravenous gammaglobulin is used to try and 'reset' the immune system. Treatment of patients is difficult given that the precise mechanisms by which tissue damage occurs is as yet unknown. We can however use information gained from the treatment of similar more common diseases to explore novel treatments for these debilitating conditions. For example, a recent therapeutic development using agents called 'biologics', which target specific pro-inflammatory molecules or their cell receptors, or the inflammatory cells themselves has been suggested for use in myositis. Pilot studies are now underway in order to determine whether controlled trials of these agents will be useful in the future treatment of myositis.

Following my Bachelor of Science degree in microbiology and biochemistry in Australia, I did an honours thesis looking at the immunology of influenza virus infection. I attained my PhD from the University of London looking at ways of measuring muscle damage in cell culture. I have published over 90 scientific papers, book chapters and other articles which have covered many different aspects of autoimmune disease. I have researched conditions such as dermatomyositis, scleroderma, vasculitis, lupus and recently rheumatoid arthritis (RA). As a result of my collaboration with Professor JCW Edwards at UCL we have pioneered a new treatment for patients with RA which has potential benefit for patients with other autoimmune diseases including myositis. I live in London with my son Toby.

3

Case
Studies

Many of the case studies appeared
in 'Living with Myositis' (2003).
However, they have all been
updated three years on and it
makes for an interesting read to
see the course of the disease.
There are also many new case
studies.

Case Studies – Dermatomyositis

Jenny
53 years old. Diagnosed aged 47. **DM**

Myositis is an illness that is very hard to diagnose and frequently misdiagnosed, but at the time this was happening to me I was angry to say the least. I felt that doctors thought I was a hypochondriac and basically an annoyance.

June 16th 1998 (A lovely sunny day) my husband escorted me to see a private rheumatologist. I was with him for about 2 hours and I think he knew already, before any tests were done, that I had dermatomyositis. I was admitted to hospital immediately and my journey began. *Isn't it great to have a name for your illness!*

A short period of optimism and relief was followed by reality.

A drip of intravenous steroids was put up. Then, 60mg of steroids were to be taken orally every day; twelve little red tablets.

'I'm sure you'll feel much stronger when this starts to work,' said my rheumatologist.

I didn't – and I stopped sleeping. My muscles had all turned to jelly and I had lost a stone in weight.

Why did I feel so bad? I still don't know – Perhaps my body has a strong aversion to drugs! Most people do feel stronger once they start steroids.

I cried buckets during those first two weeks; a mixture of the side effects of the drugs and a sort of grief. I didn't want this to be happening to me. I wanted to be at Wimbledon watching the tennis with my daughters. I just wanted to be normal. What had I done to deserve this? Had I been a bad person? Was I a bad wife, mother, daughter, sister?

The day came when I was to leave hospital and I wasn't mentally ready. I needed doctors nearby. Suppose I started to feel worse? My consultant reassured me and handed me a bag, full of drugs.

'You'll be fine. Look at your life in 10-day chunks. Every 10 days you'll realise you are just a little better than you were before. You must rest. Let your family take over the housework. Limit yourself to going up and down stairs three times a day. Oh, and you must keep out of the sun.'

'Forever?' I asked despondently.

'Yes,' he replied, 'Forever.'

I was a sun worshiper and loved getting a tan. How could I learn to like looking 'lardy'? How could this harmless pleasure be bad for me?

Ten days after coming home from hospital I felt worse.

I was told to bump up the steroids but then I started to feel even weaker.

Six weeks after diagnosis

I received a phone call from my consultant.

'Stop the azathioprine immediately. It's affecting your liver.' *Ah, so that's it. That's why I feel so lousy.* The following week I put these entries in my diary: – *Managed to walk down the garden today and sat in a chair* (In the shade of course + hat, long sleeves etc. etc.) *Managed to cut up my own dinner.*

I struggled on until early August putting up with a bangy heart, fiery arms and legs, sweats, heartburn, extreme weakness, many emotional outbursts, tears, sleeplessness and depression.

Eight weeks after diagnosis

A sticky, sweltering August continued and I began to walk a bit more but always paid for it later with fiery burning legs. I started to taper the steroids. Kind friends started to take me out for drives and I managed to do short walks around garden centres and such like. Wonderful! I was doing well.

Then BANG!

Four days after reducing to 50mg from 60mg prednisolone I was so weak that I could hardly speak, let alone walk. I was breathless, fluttery, shaky, felt sick and thought I was about to have heart failure.

I staggered to my GP.

'I'm afraid Mrs Fenton, that a very few people have problems tapering steroids. It appears that you are one of them.'

A day later my husband drove me to casualty, as I was feeling so ill. My husband went into the hospital to get me a wheelchair and I stayed lying down, in the back of the car. Suddenly there was a CRASH! A car had reversed into ours. I was too weak to do anything about it and the man drove off quickly. Two days later I managed to tell my husband who had been wondering why the front of the car was dented!

Two months passed and I felt worse than ever.

Then they found another problem. I was low on potassium. No wonder I felt so weak. Another drug to add to my list. By now I had so many drugs to take, I started a timetable.

'*Can all these drugs actually be doing me good?*' I asked myself.

Two days later, up went my temperature and I started weeing blood. (This was to be the first of many urinary tract infections (UTI's) to which I have become susceptible since being on steroids.)

Out came the emergency doctor, as it was, of course, a Saturday! (You'll probably find that most crises inevitably happen at weekends!) A course of antibiotics was prescribed. Forty-eight hours later, on my 48th birthday, diarrhoea started and I could hardly lift my head off the pillow. At 1.00am I was admitted to hospital and a drip was put up. I was so weak I couldn't even raise my arm to scratch my nose. I didn't sleep in the hospital, as I was put in a mixed, noisy ward full of very sick people, all crying out for a nurse. A tramp in the bed next to me urinated all over the floor. Later he discharged himself and in doing so, fell across my bed in his urine stained clothes.

I wretched. Maybe I was in hell.

Over the next five days my steroids were reduced and I was monitored very carefully.

I started to feel a little stronger and went home for the Bank Holiday weekend.

A bad move.

By the Bank Holiday Monday I felt my battery had finally run out and because it was a Bank Holiday we called out a private doctor, who is also a good friend, and who has always come up trumps when needed. I could tell from his face that he thought I was seriously ill and by lunchtime I was in a hospital. I stayed there for 10 days. By now I had become anaemic too! My eyes had also started to play up and were refusing to focus on long distances. Whilst in the hospital I went to see an eye specialist, (who happened to have the worst bad breath ever!) and he found nothing wrong. I can only assume that the steroids were to blame but this has never been ascertained. The inability to focus improved as I reduced the steroids but I do now have to wear glasses all the time. My eyesight deteriorated rapidly.

By the time I got home again I had reduced the steroids even further. Wow – I was doing well!

Three months after diagnosis I was feeling so well I made another entry in my diary 'A *new start*' and I felt VERY optimistic.

October came and with it my eldest daughter left home and went to university for the first time. I felt a mixture of pride and abandonment. Pride for obvious reasons and abandonment because since my diagnosis 4 months previously she had been with me every day. I was terrified to be left by myself while my other two daughters were at school and my husband at work. But I knew I had to start coping on my own and overcome this fear.

Before she went she suggested we went for a short walk. I could still only do a couple of houses up the road! We crossed the road and she took my arm. I suddenly twigged as to what was on her agenda and I froze! Her mission was to get me up our road to the local shops! This is a distance of about 20 houses and also slightly up hill!

'I can't possibly do that,' I yelled at her, 'I haven't got the energy.'

'Yes, you have,' she answered with quiet determination and off we went – VERY SLOWLY!

You can't believe how thrilled I was when I achieved this small goal. It now meant I could go shopping! During the next few weeks I went for a short walk every day. Every few days I would go a little further, until eventually I could walk for half an hour. I also took up knitting as it helped me to gain strength in my arms and hands. That year everyone got a scarf for Christmas and my great nephew got a lovely striped cardigan! OK – so it sort of fell off his shoulders - but who cares - I had made it!

Eventually I started driving again. At first I had trouble getting the handbrake off but with two hands I eventually succeeded. We also changed our big car for a much smaller one with power assisted steering. A 'must' for anyone with myositis. Being able to drive again opened up a whole new world for me.

Six months after diagnosis I had tapered the steroids quite a lot and I was walking pretty well. The New Year was a real turning point with my attitude towards the DM. I decided I had had enough of 'being ill' and consciously decided to fight it. I was going to win **not** the DM!

I was still unable to work as a teacher of English to foreign students but I busied myself doing other things. I joined a diet and exercise class in a local church hall. It was time to shed some of the weight I had gained due to the steroids. I was beginning to regain my self-esteem and became interested in clothes again. I had completely lost my sparkle during the worst part of the illness (with good reason) and had slobbed around in baggy T-shirts and strange baggy 'fatigue' trousers. Not very flattering! All my friends and family know me as being a complete shopaholic for clothes and so they knew I was getting better when I started to come home laden with carrier bags which I would try to secrete in my wardrobe, away from my husband's eye!

I helped to start a self-help group at my hospital for the rheumatology department. This has gone from strength to strength and I find it very rewarding. Lately, my friend and I have started a London Group for people with myositis (an extension of the Myositis Support Group in Southampton). This is growing so rapidly that soon we shall need a hall to hold our meetings in rather than my front room!

I had sixteen months off work and now work part-time. It can be exhausting at times and I have to pace myself. Pacing myself is something I'm NOT good at and I often suffer because of it.

I can't take the heat anymore; it's as if my thermostat has gone wrong! I am still on steroids, but a very low dose. I keep the drugs I have to take to a minimum (with my consultant's approval, of course!) and I try to look after my body as well as I can, by being careful what I eat. I avoid additives as much as I can, and get advice on vitamins and minerals that may help me. I am also teetotal. I have also recently been diagnosed as having Coeliac Disease, so that complicates things even further!

Having DM can certainly cause acute severe depression at times. I think this is quite understandable. Your life suddenly, without warning, changes. It takes time and a lot of support and understanding to come to terms with this. I urge everyone who is not coping to get help and go for counselling. Don't feel you're a failure – you're not. Try to feel reassured that not every day will be a bad day and that the depression will pass. When you have a good day – live it to the full. This doesn't mean you have to exhaust yourself. Perhaps you could do something creative. Lots of people with a chronic illness take up a craft. I took up watercolour painting, which I hadn't done since my art college days, 30 years ago!

On the negative side having myositis and being on steroids has caused my looks to change. This was particularly upsetting when I met up with an old boyfriend again and he didn't recognise me. It really rubbed it in.

My lovely long, thick, wavy hair has become thinner and I have to wear it short. My body has changed shape and is not as toned as it once was. My stomach is distended from steroid use. My skin has become thinner and rather translucent, so I tend to wear a false tan all the time. It makes me feel better. I also get very tired easily and I find it hard trying to explain to friends that I just can't stay up late any more. Sometimes I have to cancel a prior engagement at short notice as I have simply run out of steam! Because I look fine with my make-up on I think that people think I'm being pathetic. I also hate being so dependent on drugs. It's not a nice feeling.

I often feel I have had more than my fair share of suffering until I remind myself of those who are far, far worse off than I am. It helps to keep things in perspective

So what good has come from having dermatomyositis?

I have made loads of new friends. I have found out who my true friends are. I have found out what is important in my life and I strive to achieve it. I try to help others suffering with this illness and the depression that comes with it and find my new 'life' very rewarding.

Myositis is certainly no walk in the park and I am extremely fortunate that I have responded well to treatment. I have also been lucky in that I have a very caring and competent rheumatologist.

Obviously I would have preferred not to have had DM, but I did and I try to live life to the full. *Update – see 'Remission' chapter.*

Julie   DM
45 years old. Diagnosed aged 29.

Return to freedom – life with and after Dermatomyositis

This story has been written in the hope that it may give the reader inspiration and encouragement. It is a story of endurance, pain, tears, and laughter. A chapter describing a life changing experience, and living proof of the power of prayer.

September 1986 was a turning point in my life. At the time I had been working as a Hotel Manageress, enjoying the freedom of being single and I was generally, in good health, (or so I thought). However, I developed a severe sore throat forcing me to take sick leave, soon becoming dehydrated. An angry looking boil appeared on my left knee and was painful to the point that I had difficulty putting my foot to the ground.

As I became weaker, I could no longer continue living on my own and went to stay at my parent's house for some T.L.C. Things went from bad to worse as ulcers broke out all over my body. Doctors were baffled and unable to provide a diagnosis. The ulcerated rash spread to my eyes, ears and nose. I was sure it was an adverse reaction to the antibiotics.

I remember one Sunday afternoon the doctor visited me and asked me if I was willing to go into hospital for some tests. I was only too happy to oblige, not thinking for one moment that this would be my home for the next five months!

I was only in hospital about two weeks when my immune system went into reverse; my internal organs rapidly failing. I was rushed to an intensive care unit and put on a life support machine. I remained on the machine for two months with about 21 tubes coming out from everywhere. Unbeknown to myself, my parents were told by doctors every day to spend as much time as they could with me, as I might not be around in the morning. I am sure they suffered more than I did; I was certainly unaware I was so ill. 'Something' seemed to take over me.

I remember having two nurses with me all day and one by night. During the two months, I was given a tracheostomy, was linked up to a kidney machine and heart monitor and had to have surgery to remove part of my bowel, which resulted in the need for an ileostomy. The hospital also made a huge mistake in giving me a blood transfusion of the wrong group.

Whilst my family kept vigil by my bedside, the congregation of the Baptist church of which I was a member, organised a 24-hour 'prayer chain'. This meant them arranging a rota of people who were willing to pray for my family, and myself so that there were prayers being said continually.

It was through the diagnosis of a retired skin specialist that enabled doctors to begin appropriate treatment. Massive doses of steroid gave me the all too familiar moon face and swollen body, but at least it began to control the ravaging effects of the disease.

Anyone who has myositis will be aware of the pain and weakness to muscles. Immobility quickly results in muscle wastage. Not everyone thankfully will experience all the added complications I had. When I was eventually independent of the life support machine I remember having to have saline baths to dry up the rash. As the salt began to dry, the stinging was horrendous. The rash had to be dressed several times a day with a type of thin green foam, which is used, for severe burns. I must have looked like a Martian!

My body, once ballooned with steroids had now shrunk to six stone, I had lost most of my hair, but it was growing again. I was also having sight problems as retinal bleeding was diagnosed. My parents were given permission to take me out for a drive one afternoon. To see green fields and blue sky again was marvellous. At Christmas, I was allowed home for a few days. I was very weak and had to use a wheelchair, but it was great to be 'home'. I remember having to eat a pureed Christmas dinner as my throat muscles were weak and damaged by the tracheostomy, but I didn't mind. My friends and family were delighted that I was on the road to recovery, as they did not expect me to ever leave hospital. It was quite funny trying to watch an episode of Fawlty Towers on television. I had to laugh silently as the tracheostomy had damaged my voice box and I had to learn to talk all over again.

In total, I spent five months in hospital with intensive rehabilitation and therapy. I was unable to return to my own home for a number of months as I needed to be fed, washed, dressed and assisted to walk, so had to move back with my parents. It was very frustrating to have to rely on others for basic needs, especially after living an independent life and having an active career. It was hard work for my mum as she was constantly 'on the go'. She did not, I am sure, expect to be looking after a 29 year old. My mum also worked hard whilst I was in hospital trying to liaise with my mortgage lenders and utility suppliers to explain how ill I was and the reason why my bills were not being paid. A very helpful solicitor wrote letters on my behalf to stop bailiffs taking over my property.

An occupational therapist from social services visited us at home. She organised for the bed and chair to be raised and arranged for the delivery of a backrest for the bed. I couldn't help but laugh, but when the backrest arrived, it was so rusty that my mum refused to have it inside the house! We also had a home help for a while to support my mum with domestic activities. It was quite embarrassing that I had to have an ex boyfriend to lift me in and out the bath (I did wear a swimming costume though, much to his annoyance I expect!).

As you know, there is no cure (as yet), for myositis, only treatments that may slow down the disease or keep it under control. However, I believe that having a positive attitude can play a significant part in rehabilitation. When you go through something such as this, you must not give up, you need to think about your strengths and make the most of what abilities and skills you do have.

It was with this strength and determination that I agreed to continuing physiotherapy and speech therapy to enable me to regain some of my lost activities of daily living. For a time, I lost confidence in myself. I had been in a protective environment for such a long time, that the big wide world was frightening. I had to force myself to join a craft class for disabled people to get myself socialising with other people. This led on to some voluntary work opportunities with Mencap and assisting with the selling of crafts their members had produced.

Gradually my confidence and abilities returned. After about six months, I returned to my own home. For some time I still needed a lot of help for tasks of daily living and could not walk far. I wondered if I would ever get back to how I used to be. I found a lot of comfort and support from the church and God taught me to be patient and to rely on Him. Twelve months after surgery I was able to have the ileostomy reversed.

It was probably about 18 months before I felt well enough to be involved in some kind of retraining for employment. I really did not know what to do. I knew I would not have the stamina for hotel catering again. I decided to enrol on a government-funded programme and I learnt to type and use a computer. Through this I gained Pitman's and RSA qualifications. I thought perhaps that I could use this together with my hotel experience to get a job as a hotel receptionist. The agency found me a six-month's placement, meaning that I could give it a try but still retain my welfare benefits.

I found this post to be extremely boring. I was reading a book most of the afternoon! I knew I had greater potential. I spoke to my 'Project Development Officer' (PDO), stating I would like to work with disabled people and felt that because of what I had been through I could empathise and relate well to them. There was a Community Resource Centre near my home where adults with learning disabilities worked. I suggested that she try to get me a placement there. My PDO had quite a defeatist attitude. She said, 'You will never get into there, you are not qualified'. Instead, she sent me for an assessment to a college for people with disabilities. I had to do all sorts of childish tests like putting shapes in holes! I felt quite humiliated. I'd suffered a muscle wasting disease not partial removal of the brain!

This experience made me more determined than ever to do what I wanted to do. I made an appointment to visit the Community Resource Centre and the manager agreed to take me on as a volunteer. This provided a wonderful opportunity to gain not only experience, but to build up my strength and stamina. After only a few months, a temporary paid position became available. I applied for the post and got it. Twelve happy months were spent teaching independent living skills to adults with learning disabilities.

During this time, I also met my present husband. We had a whirlwind romance and he proposed two weeks after we met. I had the difficult task of explaining to him that we might not be able to have children. We were not absolutely clear about the risks to my health. Added to this, was the blood transfusion of the wrong group administered whilst in hospital. Along with the antibodies now in my blood, our blood groups were not compatible, so there was a huge risk that the baby could be born disabled. I did claim compensation for this mistake, but it could never pay for the fact that we were afraid to take a chance and made the decision not to try. On our wedding day, the Minister cried seeing me walk radiantly down the aisle.

When my temporary contract expired, I was fortunate enough to get a job as an Occupational Therapy Assistant with Social Services (1990). This led on to my employers giving me the opportunity to qualify as an Occupational Therapist. In 1993 I embarked on a four year in-service course at The University of the West of England in Bristol, whilst still working. My husband and mum were very proud to attend my graduation in 1997 at Bristol Cathedral.

My consultant was helping to wean me off steroids, but every time, we tried to reduce them I would get some kind of infection. It was an extremely slow process. In 1990, I came off them for a while, but started to get pains in my legs. However, I am now pleased to say that since July 2001, I have not been taking any medication whatsoever. I still see my consultant bi-annually for a check up, but otherwise am well. I am now working as a Senior Occupational Therapist with Social Services and get a thrill when I am able to facilitate a person's recovery.

On reflection, I feel privileged to have been through this experience. It has taught me to be patient and has made me into a better person. I have met lots of people who I would not have if I had not had this condition. I have certainly found out who my friends are. I have had to fight for what I want, and wanted to give up many times. Although my husband did not know me when I was very ill, he has been a tremendous support in the years we have been together.

I count my blessings for what I have and what I am. Without determination, self-will and love of others we are nothing. I now look forward to what the years have in store for me and remain excited in the knowledge that there is real power in prayer and that miracles did not just happen in Bible times. God bless you all.

Keep smiling.

Update

I was privileged to be asked to tell my story at the Myositis Conference in Birmingham in July 2003. During this event, the first edition of "Living with Myositis" was launched and I have had the opportunity to share it with many friends, relatives and work colleagues.

Just recently, I was feeling particularly unwell, with flu like symptoms, aching muscles and waves of extreme tiredness. With a case history such as mine, you automatically associate any illness with myositis. Oh, ye of little faith!! My doctor carried out numerous blood tests, but thankfully, all showed normal. I put it down to being over worked!

I am writing this addition to my original story during Easter 2005. The Easter story reminds me that the pain I went through was nothing compared to what Jesus himself suffered.

I am pleased to report that I have been off all medication for nearly four years and fully discharged from hospital check ups for nearly two. On the last visit to see my consultant, I presented him with a signed copy of the book, with instructions to lend it to students and any patients with myositis who might find it a source of help and support.

We should be thankful for all the work the Myositis Support Group does for all of us, for, without dedicated volunteers and fund raising, valuable research into a cure for these conditions will not materialise.

Val   **DM**
51 years old.

November 1993

Having never been a particularly sickly person – didn't get many colds or flu – I went down with a really bad bout of flu – it completely knocked me for six.

I got over it reasonably well but the following January/February I noticed that my thighs sort of ached when I stooped down – put it down to age, I thought!

Anyway, time marched on, but in the following June I developed a rash on my arms. I thought it was an allergy to conifers in the garden

when I had been weeding. I went to my GP's and was given antihista-
mines (the itching was driving me mad.) 'Come back in three days if it
doesn't improve.' – back I went – steroid cream this time – 'Come back
next week if it doesn't improve.' Back I went again! This time I saw a
young lady GP and I told her that my arm muscles were really aching
and that I found it quite difficult to hang my washing up – could the
two be linked? She looked concerned and said that she would take
blood tests, arrange for an appointment with a dermatologist and we
would go from there.

Luckily the appointment came through for the following week. So
off I trotted to see the dermatologist. When I sat down she looked concerned and asked if I had regular smear tests, carried out regular breast
checks and had I noticed any unusual lumps or bumps. Hang on a
minute – I thought I came here with itchy arms!!! I must have looked
very puzzled and so she explained to me that my blood tests revealed
that I was suffering from dermatomyositis which sometimes showed
itself when there was a hidden cancer. Well, you could have floored
me. I couldn't even say the word let alone understand the condition.
She took a skin biopsy and sent me home. I still was at a loss – more
that I could be suffering from the big C.

Anyway, I had only been home about an hour when the rheumatology department rang and said they wanted to admit me. This was
going from the sublime to the ridiculous!!

Next day off I go again – husband in tow! I was admitted and a
young registrar sat on my bed and explained that the diagnosis was
confirmed as DM, that it was an extremely serious condition and that I
would have to undergo further tests, which over the next few days I
did. Well that was the start. Obviously the drug therapy started, prednisolone first of all, several months later azathioprine and the condition stabilised. However, after several months the azathioprine wiped
out my immune system and I was prescribed methotrexate.

Over the last seven years I have had some relatively good periods
but equally some pretty miserable ones when the disease really
becomes quite active – so up go the steroids – get it stabilized – back
off the steroids for a few more months. It is like being on a merry-go-
round. At the moment, I am having a relapse so have had to triple the

normal steroid dose and now it looks like the metho-trexate is causing anaemia. Could it be back to the drawing board?

The main problem I have encountered is getting understanding. Apart from a rash on the face and hands I don't look that ill. I managed to lose all the weight I gained from taking the steroids, which has made me feel better about myself – but to put over how you feel is difficult. The worst part is that as the condition is rare, the medical profession seems to be in the dark. My consultant has told me that I can monitor my condition far better than he can. Another told me only recently 'The disease is only really active for five years.' – I told him that I had already been suffering for over seven!!

I took part in the Creatine Trial but I've no idea what I was taking – the creatine or the placebo. But it was really great to go to Dulwich and talk to the doctors and staff there who really do know what myositis is about. Obviously the Myositis Support Group is brilliant too in keeping me in touch with development and also to just know that I'm not on my own.

Still, I have never been one to give in. My philosophy is that DM will not beat me – I will beat it – I just make good use of the good days and accept the bad.

Update

Unfortunately there has not been any dramatic improvement. I have had several relapses and I have had pulse treatments, a short spell in hospital and now I am taking cyclosporine along with methotrexate and prednisolone. I feel I must rattle.

I have had to learn to live with the disease and just hope that someday (after 11 years) that I might go into remission. Every time I visit the hospital and see another new registrar they seem amazed that my DM is still active. My consultant is desperate to get me off steroids and I have managed to get down to 5mg daily but of course there are side effects. The cyclosporine has caused high blood pressure – so another tablet. The steroids have caused cataracts in both eyes which require surgery.

Last year we moved to a smaller house which has made life easier housework wise. I am fiercely independent and try to do as much as possible. Things are difficult and some tasks are impossible and then I do have to ask for help but saying that, there are still good things in my life - my wonderful family especially – so life could be worse.

Female   **DM**
77 years old. Diagnosed aged 23.

My story is not particularly remarkable, except in the fact that I have survived dermatomyositis for 53 years.

The diagnosis was made in 1948 when I was 23. First an unexplained rash on my arms and then increasing weakness. Thanks to an alert GP, in about six weeks I was at St T's hospital in London, where the disease was confirmed immediately by a consultant dermatologist, who is still held in high regard at that hospital years after his death.

At 23 I walked like an old woman and being no treatment in those days, I was prescribed complete rest and a high protein diet, including a protein supplement called Casilan. With loving care from my parents and my fiancée, I recovered sufficiently after about eight months to return to work part-time and shortly afterwards I got married.

A few years later I was back to normal, except that I did not have much stamina. This residual weakness has remained with me and has been a minor inconvenience, but often difficult to explain to people as I appeared well. I expect some people thought of me as a bit lazy as I never returned to work full time.

Ten years after the start of the illness, the symptoms returned and this time it was worse and I was admitted to St. T's hospital. Although cortisone was around by then, it was not prescribed, perhaps because it was so new. I had a muscle biopsy and various injections (vitamins) and then it was back to the high protein diet. A thought on this; when there were no effective drugs, the emphasis was on eating lots of protein. Since steroids etc. it is never mentioned, not to me anyway. I wonder why? Is it not necessary or desirable? I must ask someone sometime!

I recovered for a second time over a period of about four years. There followed a long remission of 20 years, then in 1981 it all came back and I found myself back in hospital, this time because I was so weak. It was considered that I had been 'lucky to have been let off the hook twice' so it was decided to start prednisolone and azathioprine. The improvement was quite dramatic and recovery much faster than before. I was amazed.

Since then I have been able to come off azathioprine but unable to come off drugs completely and for most of the time I have been on a maintenance dose of 5mg or 7.5mg prednisolone. I have had a couple of short flare-ups, but all controllable, touch wood!

Whilst on the subject of steroid treatment, it may be interesting for those who may not know, that it is possible to have a soluble type in 5mg tablets, which is supposed to be gentler on the stomach. I have been on these all the time and they can easily be halved to adjust the dosage.

As I have already said, I have been very lucky and every day since 1948 has been a bonus.

Since 1983, when my lovely supportive husband died, I have lived alone, with no family but many very good friends. I have always valued them and am grateful that they still keep in touch. Most of them have a great sense of humour, so we laugh a lot, which always makes me feel good. I listen to the radio and like to have cheerful music on. Of course I watch TV too, only selectively. (Too much doom and gloom at times!)

So, I've found that trying to be cheerful with other people brings out the best in them. It's not always been easy when one feels wretched, but it pays dividends. It all helps to bring about a positive mood and I'm sure that this is an aid to recovery.

The brightest spot is that there are now so many people, especially our support group, working tirelessly towards finding a cure for myositis. So much progress since 50 years ago, when it seemed that no one really cared. I am sure they did but it all seemed hopeless at the time.

Update

Since I last wrote life has, thankfully, continued to be good.

I reached the age of 80 last year. An attainment which I felt merited some celebration. The outcome was a very enjoyable informal party with twenty old friends.

I have kept well. Two minor problems have been fluid on the hip (now dispersed with physiotherapy) and mild psoriasis. I have had a heart valve condition for some years and this is inevitably increasing with age, so I get a bit breathless, but I cannot believe my luck at 80 – to have made it so far!

I am still on a maintenance dose of steroids with regular blood tests.

My good fortune also extends to wonderful friends and neighbours, who are my substitute family and every bit as caring as a real one. Some even invite me to stay for holidays.

Of course my muscles are weakening with age, but I pace myself as I have learned to do for most of my life. If one is lucky enough to be able to do this it is the key to a sort of contentment, I believe.

Richard (USA)   DM
Diagnosed aged 14.

I first became sick with dermatomyositis (DM) in the fall of 1964 when I was 14 years old. I was a reasonably good athlete before then, so I knew how it felt to have strong healthy muscles. The DM came on gradually, but it was most obvious when I tried to run a lap around the track during school. My legs felt like they had heavy bricks tied to each one and I could hardly run. The doctor diagnosed DM right away, though they had to verify it with a muscle biopsy. The only treatment at that time was prednisone (USA). I started taking 30mg/day and regained some strength, but I did not come close to my original strength. My muscles in my legs and arms also shortened some, which I have never been able to restore. For example, I cannot sit on the floor with my legs crossed because the muscles simply won't move into that position. I cannot completely straighten my arms either. Fortunately, these are only slight limitations.

Of course, I became aware of the side effects of prednisone through direct experience. After about one year I had to start wearing a back brace during the day. This was very uncomfortable, but there was no choice. I tried exercise to regain my strength but never had much success in getting stronger.

After about five years, maybe in 1970, my doctors started an experimental approach of combining methotrexate with prednisone. This combined treatment had some success. I was able to reduce my prednisone to about 10mg/day and received methotrexate injections about once a month. Within a few months of reducing the prednisone dose I no longer had to wear the back brace and have not worn one since then.

My biggest problem from the DM was itchy skin. I would spend close to an hour every day scratching my legs, back, ankles and scalp. We saw doctors for treatments, but nothing worked. This was devastating because my skin was red and torn up from scratching and there appeared to be no effective way of controlling it. I tried lots of 'remedies' for DM, herb potions, aloe vera, you name it – but none of these things did any good.

In 1978 I was very fortunate to start taking large doses of calcium ascorbate (same as vitamin C but buffered with calcium). I started the calcium ascorbate because it was recommended as a means of getting my calcium deposits (another symptom of DM) to go away. About the same time I was prayed for at a prayer meeting, which I believe was very instrumental here. Nothing happened to the calcium deposits, but within a few days the itching completely stopped! This was after fourteen years of one hour of scratching every day! This was totally unbelievable and I have a Ph.D in chemical engineering, but that's exactly what happened! I also had open sores in calcium deposits on my fingers that had not healed in three or four years. I could take a pocket knife and fish out little pieces of calcium from the sores. These sores all completely healed over in a short time. Just amazing!

I also decided that the most effective approach to gaining strength was to train the same way that athletes have to train to get stronger. I started an exercise programme inside my apartment with stretching, sit-ups, light weights and running in place. I was too embarrassed to go outside because the scratching had left my legs with red patches all over. I had to build up my endurance so that I could run in place for 20 minutes, but I was able to do it.

There were still some complications from taking the prednisone and methotrexate; the biggest nuisance being infections. I would get infections mainly at places where I had calcium deposits on my hands. Then I had to go to the doctor, get a prescription for an antibiotic, wait two or three days for the antibiotic to stop the infection, and repeat the whole process a few months later. I then decided that the long term effect of taking these drugs couldn't be good and I wanted to stop the medications and use the exercise and calcium ascorbate to maintain my strength. My doctor told me that there shouldn't be any side effects at the low dose I was taking, but he agreed to try the idea. Unfortunately you cannot just stop taking prednisone over night, so I had to gradually lower the dose, say from 10mg/day to 9mg/day – wait three months, lower another mg etc, etc. It took three years to get off the prednisone and methotrexate completely. That was about the end of October 1981 and I have not taken any prescription medications for DM since then.

I was convinced by people at work that I should start going to our employee recreation centre for my exercise programme. We had a dedicated triathlete-type guy in charge of the centre and he taught a 'healthy heart' class. He set up a personal programme for me to follow. This was around 1981. I still follow this programme three days a week. I do about ten minutes of warm up, which consists of neck circles, shoulder circles, trunk circles, short knee bends and side stretches. I then do about twenty minutes of cardiovascular exercise. Initially I was able to jog (though people watching me said I was only 'fast-walking' – it sure felt like jogging to me!) for twenty minutes and I could cover about one and a half miles. For about thirteen years I would jog in a five kilometre race with my brothers once a month. I was very slow. My fastest time was only thirty-three minutes for the five kilometres. I did the jogging until about 1997. Now I do twenty minutes on a Stairmaster machine, because my hips, knees and leg strength are not sufficient to jog. The last part of my exercise programme is about twenty-five minutes in the weight room on the weight machines. I use light weights and try to exercise my legs, arms and abdomen. In early 1997 I found that I didn't have enough strength and ability to work all day. My doctor put me on disability leave from work and I now can devote my effort to my health. I have remained fairly constant in strength and ability since 1997.

I was diagnosed with type II diabetes in 1992. I do not have to use insulin but take pills to control my blood sugar. I also tried creatine, which some studies have shown improves muscle strength in people with MS. I did not see any dramatic effect from the creatine.

I am 5ft 8in tall and now weigh about 115 pounds. My weight was probably around 130 pounds when I first got sick. It dropped about 20 pounds initially but has changed very little since. I take a pain killer when my muscles or joints hurt. I definitely recommend the calcium ascorbate for the DM. You should know within a few days, at least within a couple of weeks if it is going to help you feel stronger. You shouldn't use regular vitamin C (ascorbic acid) as even though it is a weak acid it can cause inflammation in your stomach. In addition be very careful of anything else containing acids if you have ever taken prednisone. I have not seen any side effects from the calcium ascorbate which I have taken for twenty two years. As well as providing the vitamin C it also provides valuable calcium which is definitely needed for anyone who has ever taken prednisone or other steroids

Update

I began to notice a very slow loss of strength, especially in my legs, beginning in 1994. Even though I continued my exercise program very faithfully, this slow loss of strength continued over the last ten years. My CPK values have always been slightly elevated, usually in the high 200-300 range. This indicated that my DM could still be active. I discussed possible treatments with my doctor and we agreed to try an IVig infusion. I had one IVig infusion in Jan 2005 with no side effects from the infusion but also no positive effects on my strength or muscle pain. It did lower my CPK to 56, which was my first normal value in forty years. However, the very next month the CPK was back to 290. This may be due to the short half-life of IVig inside the body (about 21days) after an infusion. In my doctor's office his colleagues had just completed a trial study using rituxan (a B-cell depletion medication) for rheumatoid arthritis patients with extremely good results. These good results, together with reported benefits of rituxan with small numbers of patients with DM, provided the incentive to try rituxan myself. I had two infusions of 1000 mg each of rituxan in April and May 2005. I had an allergic reaction during the first infusion which was controlled with Benedryl. I experienced no negative side effects from the rituxan, but I am not taking any medications that suppress the immune system so I may not be susceptible to infections as prednisone or methotrexate could cause. It is very early to expect significant results from the rituxan, but I have improved slightly in strength in my weight-training exercises and I have noticed less muscle pain. So far no change in my CPK has occurred.

John   DM
59 years old.

Dear Dermo,

I thought I would write to let you know the profound effect YOU have had on my life.

When YOU first arrived with your mate DIABETES, in October 2000 my life was OK, a bit hit and miss but OK. Then out of the blue YOU arrived, and for over a month YOU had the doctors totally confused, and my wife at her wits' end with worry. Through her persistence, the surgery sent a new doctor round and he thought he knew who YOU were. This was early evening on December 14. He phoned the L&D and I was admitted.

After lots of tests, the doctors were still not sure who YOU were. Then along came Dr S – she had a very good idea who YOU were, and after research via email to the states YOU were identified. I was then let out for Christmas, which was awful, all because of YOU. I was unable to dress myself, go to the toilet without help, I could not get off the loo. Have YOU any idea how degrading it makes ME feel? I could not feed myself, dress myself, get out of a chair without help. Even getting into bed I needed help. YOU made me dribble, which I still do. At one point, I was unable to swallow, which meant I could not eat. We missed going out with John and Wendy, and the family Christmas dinner at the Harrow had to be cancelled – all because of YOU!

Early January 2001 I had to go back to the L&D for more tests, which included biopsies to my arm and leg. After being moved from ward to ward, it was decided to let me go home until the stitches were due to come out. Later I had to go back because my leg was bleeding so badly. I was then referred to the district nurse who came every day for three weeks. As you can see so far, YOUR visit has not been welcome, but there is more.

I was then called back to the L&D and kept in. First in ward 3, then 21, then 4 where I stayed for about five weeks during which time I had more tests, x-rays, scans, pricks and pokes every day. All this while taking loads of pills, most of which I am still taking. The good news is that the tests showed that there was nothing more serious than YOU.

In ward 4 the showers did not work. I was unable to shower without help anyway. However, on Sunday 28 Jan I was allowed home for a shower. JUNE came for me, drove me home, helped me up the stairs and into the shower. The first one for four weeks – yes I stank! She got me dressed and back to the ward just in time for dinner. By the way, the hospital food was great; I have had worse at the Hilton. Then back to the routine, more x-rays, pricks and pokes, things shoved up my bum and down me throat. I was then discharged but had to go back as an outpatient every Monday. On one of these visits, Dr S said she had booked me into the CHEMO ward – PANIC– for a course of immunoglobulins. 'What' I hear you say.

The course lasted eight hours per day for five days. Each day I had nine bottles of the stuff through a canula in my hand. I had three sessions of five days over three months and a total of 135 bottles.

After the treatment, most of my hair fell out. It has now started to grow, not much but it's back.

So here we are a year on and I am still taking loads of pills, which I will be taking for the foreseeable future. Still dribbling and attending the outpatients' dept every Monday for blood tests, and having counselling, which I hope will help YOU on your way.

All in all, it has not been very pleasant having YOU around. YOU have almost cost me my business, our house, and we have not been able to go on holiday. But this year we are having one. SO UP YOURS!! YOUR visit has also taken its toll on my body. I am unable to do the things I like doing; golf, DIY, walking, even going to the toilet is not the same. I still need help dressing all because YOU have taken my muscles. I am also trying to lose weight but because of all the pills, I am not having much success. YOU have also made ME tearful, mainly from frustration. With total pissed-off-ness!

As you might have gathered by now it has not been pleasant having YOU around and the sooner YOU go the better.

Update

It has been some time since my last letter to you, so with a nudge from my friend Jenny, I thought it was about time I let you know how things are progressing.

Well here we are five years down the line and sad to say you are still here. Not as bad as you were but still here. I am still going to the hospital on a weekly basis, still taking loads of pills and potions.

Because of you damaging my leg muscles, I was unable to walk with aids. This in turn caused blood clots; one of which found its way to my left lung. I was not aware of it, I just thought it was a shortage of breath. Then I drove into town to meet June. When she came out of the shop I was slumped over the wheel. She got help and they got me into the passenger seat. She then took me straight to the doctors. He called me some very strange medical names and called an ambulance but it was quicker for June to take me to the hospital, where they were waiting for me. Yes you guessed it, more pricks and pokes. Every day I had an injection in my belly. It left me with an enormous bruise. I looked like I had done ten rounds with Mike Tyson. Two months later I left hospital clutching yet more bags of pills. Then came the warfarin and weekly co-ag checks. The car knew its way to the L&D by itself. From then on things have just plodded along. I was then told to have an EMG test on my legs, which are still very painful, so along I went. This guy stuck needles in my thighs, wiggled them about and said 'there is no sign of DM'. I am not going to tell you what I said!! I then had a visit from the Department of Work and Pensions doctor. He did some tests (he came when I was having a very bad day) the outcome of which was in my favour. I got my benefits.

It is now May 2005, and because of you I have lost the business, the car, our nice house and most of my health. All in all you have done a good job.

David   **DM**
45 years old.

My story is a positive one, due mainly to the prompt diagnosis and action by my GP.

I had been suffering for several months from tiredness, general weakness in my arms and legs and itchy skin. My symptoms gradually got worse, to the point where I could hardly hold my arms above my head and it was becoming impossible to work efficiently (I am a builder). When it reached the point that I had to lift my legs in the car manually, I decided to visit my GP.

At first my doctor was treating me for arthritis and a possible allergy. The latter for which, he made me an appointment at St. T's Hospital. My wife was insistent, after this diagnosis, that my condition was not caused by arthritis, as the problem was obviously, in my muscles, not my joints.

I took the tablets that I had been given for the arthritis and my condition deteriorated. My skin became much worse and my eyelids became swollen. Consequently, on my next visit to the doctor, as soon as he saw me, he said that my skin condition was definitely NOT an allergy. He took some blood for testing and put me on a low dose of steroids.

On receipt of my blood results, my GP told me that he suspected I had dermatomyositis and upon which then acted with great speed. By the end of morning surgery he had phoned my wife to confirm an appointment at G's Hospital the following day. My wife, in the meantime, had looked up the condition in a medical book and was by now panicking!

On visiting G's Hospital the next day, I was amazed when I was told that I would have to be kept in for further tests and I was also transferred to St. T's hospital. My GP's diagnosis was confirmed and I was then given numerous tests to try to locate the cause, of which one was never found. I was put on high dose steroids and also skin treatments. After a 10-day stay in hospital, I returned home, still on the steroids and also cyclosporin. This was in November 1998.

Since my release from hospital, I have been treated as an outpatient at G's Hospital by Prof. H. My condition has gradually and slowly improved and my medication decreased until it was eventually stopped.

My dermatomyositis is now in remission and I am leading a fit and healthy life, visiting the hospital at three monthly intervals to be monitored.

As you can see, mine is a totally positive story and I hope it will encourage others.

Postscript

My DM returned three or four months ago, for which I was hospitalized for two days in an effort to try to get on top of the condition before it worsened. I was put on steroids again and they are gradually being reduced. Hopefully, this will have the effect of the condition going back into remission. Only time will tell!

Update

Since my second bout of dermatomyositis and subsequent return to medication, my symptoms have been kept under control. However, although in apparent 'remission' my consultant is reluctant to withdraw the steroids at present and I am currently in the process of lowering the dosage very gradually with the hope that the symptoms will not return.

My quality of life is good and for fellow sufferers out there, there is light at the end of the tunnel!

Seema   **DM**
34 years old. Diagnosed aged 26.

Suddenly I burst out crying! I couldn't tie my shoelaces! In fact that wasn't the only thing. Over the past few weeks, waking up in the morning and the thought of having a shower filled me with dread. Just moving my hands was tiring and I couldn't keep them up in the air for more than a couple of seconds. Combing my hair was also very tiring. All these normal, everyday activities had become extremely difficult and I remember trying to accomplish them as quickly as possible.

I realised that that was the first time I had actually cried in public. I had been secretly worried and scared up until now but didn't want it to show. After all, I was only 26 and quite fit and healthy, and I hadn't seen a doctor in six years – it didn't make sense! Maybe part of me thought it was probably something silly and if I ignored it long enough it would eventually go away.

It had all started around Christmas 1994, initially feeling very run down and tired – almost like flu without the cold. I took a couple of weeks off work to rest. The doctor thought it might be yuppie flu and prescribed ibuprofen. This did not help so I decided I should go back to work. Monday morning, after an hour working on the computer I couldn't sit up anymore – I let my head flop onto my arms and rested it on the desk. Then there was the rash, which had initially started just before Christmas 1994, on my left cheek, then throughout January had slowly appeared on the right cheek and then onto the bridge of my nose – almost in a 'butterfly' pattern. I had tried Chinese herbal medicine – cut out dairy, applied herbs etc, but it didn't have any effect on the rash. As January rolled into February, I seemed to have less and less energy to do anything and my appetite was diminishing each day. There was just this constant aching, not pain, just aching and feeling lethargic – I just could not bring myself to do anything – I just felt like I needed to lie down all the time and sleep or rest. This was very unlike me. My mum tried to massage my arms to ease the aching, but this only seemed to make things worse.

The following morning, I could barely move. My arms and upper body was completely swollen. That morning I was admitted as an emergency to my local hospital. Despite several prior requests to the GP to do more blood tests, I was ignored for the diagnosis was 'yuppie flu' and ibuprofen was the best medicine.

20 February 1995 – '... Had to do tests... staying in for a while...' I can't remember how I took all this in at the time, except that what was being said didn't make sense The words were going round in my head and all I wanted to do was go home and wake up from this bad dream.

The next significant time was the seeing the doctor and being told (in summary):

'Polymyositis!... CK approximately 12000, should be under 200... staying in for a few months... '

Something the doctor said triggered something inside of me. I thought right, I'll show you, I'm going to get rid of this thing and be out of here a lot sooner than you think!

At the hospital I wasn't able to do anything alone, my mother had to do everything for me, from feeding to bathing. It was like being a 'big' baby! The hardest part was losing my independence and being totally dependent on someone for everything including using my finger to remove an eyelash from under my eye. The medicine didn't seem to take effect straight away, only after two weeks did the swelling reduce, and that amazingly, it did overnight. Over the next few weeks it became apparent that damage had been done to the torso and upper legs. Walking was difficult as well as getting up from chairs and beds; in fact the lower the chair, the harder it was to get up. Things did improve but as my walking became better, I found myself unable to swallow any foods at all. The epiglottis (the little flap at the back of your throat, which helps pass food down to the throat) had been affected. This meant two weeks on a drip for a liquid feed as well as loss of some speech. I remember having to tilt my head a particular way in order to enable myself to say certain words correctly.

With all this going on, the support, prayers and love from family and friends was enormous and I'm sure it contributed greatly towards a speedier recovery. One thing I didn't want to accept was the word incurable. I adopted the habit of saying the following affirmation every day – whether I believed in it or not and whether I felt like saying it or not:

'Miracles happen every day, I go deep within to dissolve the pattern that created this, and I now accept a divine healing' – ('You Can Heal Your Life' by Louise Hay).

Although at times I felt scared and frustrated, there was a strong feeling inside me that told me that I would be 100% fine. However family did not have the same insight and insisted that I see a number of spiritual healers. I had always believed in GOD (or source or a higher being – whatever you want to call it) but almost in the background, but at that time I was about to realise the spiritual side of myself more at the forefront. I agreed to see one healer and was able to leave the hospital once a week to see him; I really didn't expect anything from it, except that I would make my parents feel better. Amazingly however, the healing helped me towards a much faster recovery.

One incident I remember vividly was at a point when I had had difficulty with my hip and was not allowed to walk in case of causing further damage. Time had passed and I felt that it had improved, however I had to wait for an assessment before I got the go ahead to start walking. I remember having a dream in which I felt I was floating slightly above the ground (almost hovering) and finding myself in a place in which I was completely surrounded by rays of white light. It felt really warm and I knew it was healing me. I felt and knew there was a presence of someone else there but could not actually see anyone. I was being bathed in this gentle white light and the feeling was that of pure bliss, peace, happiness… yet those words only described the tip of what it was like. There was no one or even a few words that could describe it all. I felt so free – no baggage, no worries, just pure bliss. I am sure it must be where people go when they die, because strangely I felt so 'at home', and maybe a little part of me didn't want to leave at all.

The next day I had my assessment and I was able to walk a lot better and show that I was certainly on the road to recovery. My progress continued and I left the hospital. After all I had a party to attend, to celebrate my birthday and say thank you to all those who had helped me along the way – family, friends, doctors and nurses. I had organised it whilst being in hospital, with help from friends of course.

It had been seven whole weeks, it wasn't easy by any means but strangely I felt the happiest I have ever felt. At times I felt as if the middle of my chest had a white heart that was just radiating rays of white light filled with love all around me. I only needed four hours of sleep, and also felt more psychic, even a few conscious levels higher if that makes sense – like being a little higher up the mountain of life and getting a broader perspective of the world below – effects of prednisolone – apparently not! Maybe because I was unable to use the energy physically, it became mental energy! I had become so determined to be independent and not count on anyone for anything that it seemed as if this whole experience came about to teach me humility. When you have to rely on someone else for every single thing, it really does make you humble! Still, I can truly say, with my hand on my heart, that I do not regret a single moment of it.

A year and a half later, 4 July 1996 I was off all medication. I had done well and recovered a lot sooner than anyone (but me) had expected. It was a one in a million chance of getting the illness and a one off… or so I was told and so I believed!

January 2003

Two relapses later.. I have again completed all my medication (six months ago) for the third time. Each time was a slightly different case with signs of both poly and dermato myositis; I knew the starting signs and picked up on it happening quickly. Each time was much harder and I had to dig a lot deeper to find the strength to battle this thing. Each time was also different, and this last time I was on a lot more medication for a longer period of time. I didn't however, try and take shortcuts or reduce doses faster than I was advised; I had experienced the negative effects of doing this (when I thought I was being clever and knew best) – in the long run you only ended up staying on the drugs for a longer time! Physically I had put on the most weight ever – if the moon face had got any bigger, I think I would have burst!

I did start to question why it kept on happening, especially since it was meant to be a one off. What was the pattern and how could I break it? I have always read many self-healing books throughout the years, Louise Hay, Deepak Chopra, but one that struck me the most this last time was *'The Journey'* by Brandon Bays. I definitely believe it played a huge part in my recovery.

Well I truly hope I have broken the pattern and that there is no next time. I hope you too find your way back to good health.

Update

A minor relapse in December 2003 prompted me to once again make changes to my lifestyle and nutrition. I attended a naturopathy and yoga centre in India for a few weeks, which was extremely beneficial in cleansing and calming mind, body and spirit. Whilst there, I was introduced to the book "The pH Miracle" by Dr Robert Young – which I believe is the breakthrough for the cause of the majority of diseases. On my return, I put its principles of a more alkaline diet into practice, continued the yoga and also practiced "The Journey" by Brandon Bays. I was fortunate enough to maintain a more balanced lifestyle leading to a good resulting bone density scan and attaining a minimum level dose of prednisolone.

I have come to realize that it is a continual process of self monitoring and improvement in a holistic way, to maintain good health. In October 2004, to our surprise and delight I discovered I was pregnant and right now, I am looking forward to the arrival of a little bubba at the end of June 2005 – 6 week's time! As that new relationship starts, I hope that this old 'relationship' with dermatomyositis comes to a final end!

Seema had a beautiful baby daughter who is absolutely gorgeous. Mother and daughter are doing well.

Cary (USA)   DM
45 years old. Diagnosed aged 35.

Late one morning in January 1992 I was walking my son David to kindergarten when I noticed his jacket was unzipped. I knelt down, zipped it up and started to stand up. Started only, I couldn't stand up for my life. A normal person would have been scared. I just figured I needed a bit more exercise or maybe go on another diet.

I was 35, worked half time at the local hospital in the pharmacy. I walked an hour five or six times a week and swam laps when I didn't walk. I was healthy. Well, except for this mildly annoying rash I had on my hands, which a co-worker had noticed back in July. And I had cut back on my work schedule because I just couldn't get caught up on my rest. It was certainly hard being a working mom.

The next day I had an appointment with a dermatologist who was to look at that annoying rash. She took one look at my hands and asked, 'Have you experienced any muscle weakness at all?'

'Well, yes,' I said, 'Why?'

She said I had the classic symptoms of dermatomyositis.

That was my introduction to the mad, mad world of myositis.

I have lived nine years with this disease, so far. I have learned so much. Not the usual things: friendships, sunsets, the like. Other things in life had taught me that. I have learned to be weak, to let my husband and kids not just help around the house but run the house. I have learned that there are at least five different ways to fold towels. It's also OK not to fold them at all. No one is going to die if they have to eat canned chilli for dinner three nights running. Whether I'm sick or well, my husband is never going to clean off his dresser and that's just the way it is. Life, in other words goes on.

I'm stronger now, in remission, but still the first thing I'm asked by someone who hasn't seen me in a while is, 'How's that thing you have?'

The answer depends on a lot of things. Can I stand up by myself? Can I still tie my shoes? Is that one stubborn patch of purple skin rash still gone?

That thing is losing, I am winning. I'm doing well.

Faint Whisper

I was walking along the mountain of life, when
suddenly the ground gave way. Next thing I knew I was
hanging by a branch of a tree growing out of the side
of a cliff. I heard a whispered, 'Let go.'
A pastor came by and looked at me over the cliff
'Greeting, sister! How can I help you?' 'I'm stuck,'
I told him, 'here on this cliff.' 'Jesus is the
answer,' he replied, 'I will pray for you.' I heard
a whispered, 'Let go.'
A doctor came by, 'How can I be of help?' she asked.
'I'm stuck,' I said, 'here on this branch.' 'We'll do
some tests and try some medicine.' 'Let go,' came the
faint whisper.
A friend came by, 'How can I help?' she asked. 'I'm
stuck,' I said through my teeth, 'here on this cliff.'
'I'm here for you,' she said. A faint voice
whispered, 'Let go.'
Then I was alone. 'God!' I yelled. 'Where are you?
I'm stuck here on this cliff. Jesus is the answer,
medicine is the answer, friends are the answer. BUT
I'M STILL STUCK!'
I reasoned, I thought, I sought answers to my dilemma.
Nothing I could think of got me off my cliff.
Still the quiet voice, 'Let go.'
The day came when I had no help, no answers, no ideas,
no more life. I let go.
God took me in His quiet hands and gently
put me back on the mountainside.

by Cary

Update

The purple patch is missing in action so I'm still winning this war. The
child whose jacket I knelt to zip up is six feet tall and almost out on his

*own. He, my husband and our daughter all can clean, cook and do
laundry without turning anything pink or shrinking anything. We've survived quite nicely, though no one can tolerate canned chili any more.*

*However, they all still watch me carefully, see me as delicate, put
out a hand to help me up and over whatever may be in my way.
Scars, as it were, but hidden. We're like mended furniture, stronger
where the glue is but with the memory of being broken.*

*I've started walking again and have finally lost all my "prednisone
weight". I work full time. I've learned to live just today, completely
trusting God that I will still have strength and health tomorrow.*

Female   **DM**
75 years old. Diagnosed aged 67.

This began for me in 1995, with a small irritable lesion on my right
shoulder blade, which did not respond to local applications. I was
referred to a dermatologist who arranged a biopsy with the resulting
diagnosis of Lupus Erythematosis. Some months later I suddenly felt
unwell and found I had great difficulty climbing a flight of steps. This
was followed a few weeks later by gross swelling of the eyelids. It was
just my luck that day to find that the doctor on duty was the new
trainee to the practice! However, help was at hand and I found myself
admitted to hospital where a dermatologist decreed that the label was
now dermatomyositis and that it would be at least two years before I
would feel better! He was not wrong!

Then I went through the whole episode of purple eyelids, losing
frontal hair and the skin from my neck to knees becoming red and sore
– particularly over my knuckles which cracked easily and did not
respond to any local application. At one point my backside was so sore
I could barely sit! A locum registrar suggested I apply steroid cream
and wrap up in cling film! I ask you! That is about the most difficult
portion of the anatomy to apply a dressing in an ambulant patient! I
was on 20mg of prednisolone daily, with the addition of azathioprine.

I asked the consultant if he saw many like me, but I was the only one.
Having by now read as much as I could lay my hands on, I felt that I
needed a more knowledgeable opinion, so I asked my GP to arrange for
me to be seen in London. Many months elapsed before funding was

approved and an appointment was forthcoming, but I eventually took the train to the big city. After being sandbagged into position so that the muscles in my thigh could be studied (MRI scan), I was assessed for muscle strength in the physiotherapy department. I felt as though I was in the electric chair! I then had more blood tests and a muscle biopsy.

On reflection I think by this time I was probably over the worst and was gradually returning to normal. I'd had to wear wigs for over a year and when my hair eventually grew again it came back dark after having been pure white for many years.

I had to agitate with my GP to have a bone density scan and unfortunately, after all those years on steroids, a moderate degree of osteoporosis was confirmed.

Recently (May 2001) my back has developed some itchy areas again and my hair is once again breaking off.

Am I off on the same trail again?

This proved to be a flare-up – treated promptly by my GP with 40mg prednisolone daily plus azathioprine. It settled after three months. Steps, stairs and low chairs continue to be a problem but otherwise I am well.

Update

In August 2003 I had a sudden onset of extreme exhaustion with heavy aching limbs. This time, apart from hair loss my skin was not affected. I was put back on prednisolone and azathioprine for six months and I slowly began to feel 'like myself' once more. When my hair started growing again I knew I was over this attack. But I think that each time leaves me with more impaired muscle strength. However, I am now well, remembering to slap on the factor 30 (adding colour tint to reduce the pallor!) and I always wear long sleeves. I'm still looking for a flattering hat though!

Anne   **DM**
49 years old.

My experiences of life with Dermatomyositis

In April 1987, in fact on Maundy Thursday, I had a total hysterectomy, retaining both ovaries. Everything went according to plan. I initially felt very well and after a couple of weeks in hospital (during which I celebrated my 34th birthday) I went home.

At the beginning of May, my husband, two children and I spent a weekend at a caravan in Much Wenlock, Shropshire belonging to friends, as I did not yet feel up to travelling too far. It was a bank holiday weekend as I remember, and (unusually for a bank holiday!) it was quite sunny but not too hot. I sat outside for a while and before long noticed a slight rash on my arms. Of course I did not think too much of it and if anything, attributed it to either the trauma of the hysterectomy itself on my body or to the drugs I had been given during the operation and afterwards. I wonder now if it was in fact dermatomyositis, briefly raising its ugly head for the first time.

I had no more symptoms however, until the following May when we visited Turkey for the first time. The weather was wonderful and of course I did a lot of sunbathing, slapping on a high factor sun cream and wearing a hat. Always an adventurous family, we hired a car and went exploring for the second week, travelling into central Turkey and to Istanbul before returning to our base and it was during this week that I began to notice a rather strange rash on my forearms and cheeks. The rash was bright red and was raised, rather like small blisters, particularly on the arms, but thankfully it neither itched nor was it sore. If anything, it tingled when I touched it. I hated it though, as it was so obvious and looked as though I had not used any sun protection! Could this have been another early 'outing' for dermatomyositis? We have been back to Turkey at least once a year since, in fact almost twenty times, and, touch wood, I have never suffered this phenomenon again.

Nothing more out of the ordinary happened until November 1994, when colleagues at work noticed a rash on my arms. I suspected it to be German measles, and knowing that the wife of one of my colleagues was pregnant, I went to see my GP the next day. German Measles was ruled out; however this did not explain the rash and signalled a period of about seven months of going backwards and forwards to the surgery without a diagnosis.

In February 1995 my husband and I began training with the British Sub Aqua Club (BSAC), although I have to say I was a little embarrassed as by then I had the archetypal dermatomyositis 'face', with what could have been taken for a lupus 'butterfly' across my eyes. I should not have worried though, as they all accepted me for myself, not what I looked like. During this period my work colleagues, trying to be helpful, suggested that perhaps I was allergic to my facemask or the water in the swimming baths. Talk about clutching at straws! I continued to work as an Administrative Assistant with the Youth and Community Education Service of Staffordshire County Council although by now I was constantly feeling ill and looking terrible! I am normally a fairly confident person and will 'stare anybody out', but I found myself avoiding other people's gazes when out and about and walked along looking at the floor. I wanted to explain to everybody that this was not the normal me, that I had some sort of allergy or illness making me look this way. I also fell over a few times in the centre of town; once coming out of a pub although I swear that I had had lunch and not a drink! Even worse, once by a very handsome young man, who gallantly helped me up and asked if I was OK. I said I was, thanked him and walked off as if I always had blood trickling from my knee. Oh the mortification!!

After about six months, as my normal GP was not available, I had an appointment with a different GP at my surgery who thought I might have lupus. He explained briefly what this was, as I had not heard of it and said that he would arrange a consultation with a dermatologist. As my husband and I have medical insurance, I arranged to see a consultant dermatologist privately.

After examining me and asking me a few questions, Dr H recognised dermatomyositis straight away, but performed a biopsy to be quite sure. He also asked me about different things that I had not realised were connected to the disease; such as pain in my thighs when I went down stairs. It was such a relief to know what was wrong with me and I had the feeling that everything would be back to normal very shortly – until he told me that it was a chronic disease. I asked him about the prognosis; he said that the disease was so rare it was not possible to say, but that with the proper medication the disease could be managed. He prescribed a high dose of steroids (prednisolone) and I made another appointment for three weeks time, as we were going back to Turkey that week. It shows my naivety as I thought that when the steroids ran out, I just stopped taking them. Dr H must have told me about the dangers of this at the consultation, but I obviously did not take it on board. I stopped taking the prednisolone on Friday and was not seeing Dr H until the following Monday when – boy! – was I ill over the weekend! We were having a barbecue on the Sunday with our family, but I spent the day in bed and hardly remember anything at all about that day. I have never repeated my mistake again!!

On the Monday, Dr H confirmed the diagnosis and suggested I transfer back to the NHS as it was a chronic illness. I believe that this was very professional on his part, as he could have been laughing all the way to the bank on my illness! I will always be grateful to him for that. Unfortunately, he told me that I had to give up Scuba as diving and steroids don't mix! They take a year or two to leave your system and by then you are probably taking them again so it's a vicious circle.

Not long after this I became so ill that I was forced to take time off from work. In fact it was not until September 1996, thirteen months later, that I returned to work. However, that is jumping the gun. I found that I was on a never ending treadmill of visits to the hospital, as besides seeing Dr H every couple of weeks, I was seeing other consultants in other disciplines to rule out any underlying cancers or other diseases. I had test after test, including a trip to Stoke on Christmas Eve 1996 to have electrical tests on my muscles, which confirmed the diagnosis.

As I had been suffering from extremely swollen ankles, I also needed to visit the nuclear medicine department at our local hospital, where they injected an isotope into my big toe, then checked its progress through the veins. This showed up that I had lymphodema, which meant visits to the Lymphodema Clinic in Whittington near Lichfield and wearing knee high, toeless support socks. I even have to wear two socks on each leg when flying, oh well its quite fashionable now with all this worry about DVT! And I must admit I do not wear them every day; (I think its about seven months since I last wore them, as my ankles are not too bad. Ssh! Don't tell them at the clinic!!). I continued my six-monthly visits there until last autumn and now only need to see them if I think I really need to. I'm still supposed to wear the socks though!

I really suffered that summer of 1995, which you may remember was a heat wave. The steroids seemed to make the heat worse, so to help I had my hair cut fairly short (not a good idea with a 'moon face' caused by the prednisolone). I must have put on about three stone in weight and I now hate looking at holiday photos from that summer – what with the extra weight, redness and moon face yuk!! My family will not let me throw them away though, as they say that it was still part of my life. When I walked any distance, it felt as though I had knitting needles on my knees pointing up into my thigh muscles, so that every step was agony. Dr H tried various immunosuppressants, including cyclosporin, which affected my liver so I had to come off that pronto! Over time, with trial and error, we found that methotrexate was the one that suited me most.

As I have said previously, I returned to work thirteen long months later, having slowly weaned myself off the prednisolone. I still had to see Dr H regularly and also Occupational Health, but I enjoyed being back at work. Alas I only managed just over a year before I had to be off work again and this time Occupational Health suggested that if work share was not suitable, (which it wasn't – I couldn't say that I'd be well on say, Monday afternoons and ill Wednesday mornings so it would not be fair to the other person), then it would be best to take early retirement. After checking my options, I agreed that this was the best way forward and became a pensioner at 44!

Last year my husband and I celebrated our 30th (Pearl) Wedding Anniversary (yes – we married young!) He has been an absolute rock throughout my illness; he is so supportive. He does all the cooking and helps out as much as he can when I am ill, despite having health problems of his own. To celebrate our anniversary we travelled to Kathmandu, where we took a sightseeing flight past Mount Everest, then travelled for three weeks around India, stopping in the best hotels, then a week in the Maldives, followed by a couple of days in Dubai. My leg gave way coming down a flight of steps at Dubai airport and although I didn't actually fall, it severely dented my confidence about steps. As we live in a bungalow I don't get much practice at home!

Although I do have a flare up every now and then, I try not to let this disease have all its own way. I am currently on methotrexate, and touch wood, have just a few symptoms. A slight rash (particularly on the elbows where it has NEVER disappeared), occasional tiredness, weakness in my legs, particularly coming down stairs and a slight problem with swallowing, plus an awful backache! Nowadays I know when I am going to have a flare up and so I am better armed to fight it. I am still seeing Dr H regularly, about every five weeks, but if an appointment is not due when I have a flare up I telephone his secretary and he either adjusts my medication over the telephone or sees me earlier.

At the time of writing, I have recently had an MRI scan on my thigh muscles, which came back OK and am waiting for appointments with Ear Nose and Throat and a Speech Therapist concerning the swallowing problem. I like to think that I have a positive attitude, although it is very hard sometimes, especially when I have to go back on steroids (Dr H knows I hate them so he tries his best to keep me off them as long as possible).

Update

I have continued to see my consultant regularly, usually every twelve weeks, and have 'kept taking the tablets' (mainly methotrexate) regularly. I had a liver biopsy earlier this year to see if the methotrexate was damaging my liver. Luckily, I am OK.

I have had a few 'flares' but luckily these have only been minor. With experience I know when a flare is coming on so I'm able to stop it in its tracks. So far I have managed to stay off steroids!

Perhaps the best 'medicine' I have is our beautiful Staffordshire Bull Terrier, Tosun, who at the time of writing is nine months old. Living in the country, I have tried to take him for regular short walks locally for at least five days a week since he was old enough to be walked. We rest a lot (well, there are a lot of interesting 'sniffs' for him!!) and have fun! My husband takes him for a couple of longer walks a day, and if I'm feeling well I sometimes join them.

I have found that these regular walks have really strengthened my legs. I am finding it a lot easier to come down steps.

The future beckons!

Female   **DM**
45 years old. Diagnosed aged 35

No one person is alike. Seven years ago my illness presented itself a few weeks before my 36th birthday, although by the time I reached 36 I felt like 90! My symptoms appeared over a few weeks, whereas I

found out later that in most cases it commences over months and it is
as the doctors look back and put all the symptoms together that they
come up with a diagnosis.

　I started off with about twelve ulcers around the edge of my tongue,
which lasted just over a week. About the same time I was finding
myself getting tired doing things that I would normally do easily. My
muscles started aching in my thighs, like a pulled muscle, but it was
especially painful when climbing stairs. Instead of getting better as I
would have expected after a virus or pulled muscle, it became worse.
I found it a struggle to walk to the school with my three-year old twin
boys to pick up my four and three-quarter-year old daughter. I often
used to phone my husband to shut our shop and drive to the school
for me and drop her back as I did not feel able to go that day. I think
he used to think that I was putting it on. I did not look ill. I could only
take the dog around a quarter of the field behind our house before
having had enough.

　Eventually I needed help to get out of the car. I also used to get stuck
if I stooped down. I had to make sure that I was somewhere that I could
pull myself up with my arms! My legs just did not have the strength to
do it. My husband had to make sure the boys were dressed before he
left, as my arms were also weak and became tired when extending them
to do anything. As I am a registered nurse, I realised that something
odd was going on. It felt like climbing Mount Everest when going to the
surgery which was not a great distance away. I did not feel safe driving,
as I would have been incapable of making an emergency stop. My GP
was taking blood for tests such as glandular fever and arthritis. He eventually sent me by ambulance to the nearest general hospital eleven
miles away, after he attended me on a home visit. By this time I could
hardly climb the stairs. I dreaded the thought of going into hospital,
being a nurse, but it had got to the stage that something needed to be
done.

　My friend that day had looked after the children for me. She was
and is the best friend. She still had my three and her two children, aged
between four and three-quarters and one, nearly three weeks later, six
days a week. My husband works alone in our shop. Eventually, social
services stepped in. My friend was able to register quickly as a child
minder and looked after my children on weekdays. Our parents would

travel from Guildford, two hours away, every weekend, taking it in turns, alternate weekends, to help out. The worst thing about it all was that I felt like an awful mother. It affected one of the twins especially. It must have seemed like I'd disappeared. I felt much better knowing they were with someone they knew.

I had had a small malignant melanoma removed five months previously. The doctors were all asking questions about this. I used to think that I would not live long. I thought that I would never see the children grow up. Being a nurse made it worse. A little knowledge is a bad thing. I had not heard of dermatomyositis. I found it hard not knowing about the disease and what to expect. It was rare enough that my nursing friends did not know much about it either, except one paragraph that was not very hopeful in a nursing textbook. The doctors were saying that you were more likely to have the illness after having cancer, and I was sitting there putting two and two together and making three for the first week. It did not help the fact that it was Easter and everything was shut down for a long weekend and most of the consultants were away!

After Easter my case was then passed on to a very nice consultant neurologist. He told me a great deal about the disease. He had had a lot of experience of dermatomyositis and polymyositis in a previous job, and had referrals to the unit he was working in from all over the country. He said that the textbooks ought to be re-written, and that having cancer as a pre-disposing factor was not true. Knowing that that was not part of the trouble made a big difference to me. He outlined the investigations and treatment needed. There was only one thing that he said that did not work out right for me. I was told that diagnosis was often confirmed better on muscle biopsy. It could be diagnosed when having an electromyogram (EMG), but this was not so conclusive, and having seen these as a student nurse, I was glad that the biopsy was the first choice. I went to theatre and had a small piece of muscle taken from my thigh under local anaesthetic, but as I said before everybody is different! I think it is because I am a nurse – this came back negative! I then had to have the EMG anyway, which involved testing different muscle sites by inserting needles and recording muscle activity by sound. The consultant carried this out himself, which cheered me up a bit, as I was not looking forward to it!

However, it was worth it as he was able to make a confirmed diagnosis in order to start treatment. (Apparently the sounds made are similar to an aeroplane or motorcycle taking off! They sounded to me like an untuned radio!)

The treatment consisted of intravenous prednisolone initially of 500mg daily over three days. I then started to have oral prednisolone of 60mg daily and azathioprine 50mg. Prednisolone is a steroid, and azathioprine is a cytotoxic immunosuppressant, which both have side effects. I was asked by one of the nurses if I minded taking them, but I was grateful to do something to make me feel better. The consultant told me that the treatment would take about two years, depending on how I responded. It involved reducing the dosage of the tablets over the weeks, usually weekly. I immediately felt a lot better after the first few days, but the first time the tablets were reduced I felt like I had gone back to square one again. I eventually got used to this pattern of two steps forward and one back when reducing the medication. And true enough I was taking the medication almost two years to the day before I was able to stop them. However, initially after two to three weeks of treatment when the tablets were reduced I noticed that my swallowing was affected, but this soon passed after staying on the dose that I was on for slightly longer than intended.

Apart from cringing, having to be a patient, (I still cringe now at the thought of it!) I coped with it with the help of my own good friend, who had the children, my parents, my husband's parents and my nursing friends and colleagues. They cheered me up no end. My boss, the night sister (I worked night duty around the children) was smashing, helping with my washing, peeling fruit in the early days. I found that it was hard lifting cups to my lips, using a knife and fork, and turning magazine pages because of the damage to my muscles. She would visit me almost every day even when she was in the middle of her four night's work. And of course working night duty normally, there was always someone I knew to talk to even during unsociable hours when I could phone work! The prednisolone side effects also gave me a type of jet lag, where I could not sleep after 02.00 hrs. The girls would try to have someone to visit me most days, as my husband was quite tied up with the business and the children, and did not get to visit much except Sundays.

After three weeks in the general hospital, I spent three weeks under the care of my GP in the community hospital where I worked. Both the male and female wards wanted to have me back and that made me feel special. The male ward had nicer side rooms and a joined toilet, so I was installed in there. I was allowed to get away with lots of things, like visiting other departments and seeing everybody, going down to coffee with the nurses. My GP was great and visited me nearly every day, even if it was a social visit. However, I was still often extremely tired and needed to rest quite a bit. I enjoyed a couple of weekend leaves to go out with the family, but boy was I glad to get back to the hospital too! I also had support from the playgroup leaders who would help my husband by having the boys fifteen minutes earlier than the start of playgroup so he could open his shop on time. You find you have a lot of people rally round to do things for you if they can.

Having had dermatomyositis I have a much different perspective on life. I no longer worry about the dust; instead I will do something else, such as a bike ride or play a board game with the children. The feelings I had of not seeing the children grow up have not left me and I enjoy (almost!) all the time I spend doing things with them. I appreciate having returned back to near normal, although I still find repetitive movements tiring, such as climbing lots of stairs or cleaning windows. I am very aware of all the people who are unable to do this. Some illnesses are even worse than myositis and you do not recover from them even a little. It has made me appreciate life and how mortal we are. I think being a patient has also made me a more understanding nurse.

Update

I can't believe that it is now 10 years since I developed dermatomyositis. When I read the Myositis Support Group newsletter, I feel very lucky to have been able to stop steroids and azathioprine after only two years, as many people they need to keep taking a maintenance dose to keep their symptoms under control.

Although my consultant could not guarantee that I would never get it back, he said that as I responded so well to the treatment, he felt confident that it may not return, but that if it did then I would just start straight away on the same regime as before.

My memories of the early stages now seem a dream. I cannot believe that I needed a neighbouring patient's zimmer frame in order to reach the toilet one night (the nurses were having a horrendous night, and I did not want to bother them!), and that the walls were really useful to lean on when you needed to get anywhere!

I no longer need the walls to get about! I have found repetitive movements a bit of a problem over the years since. Walking up steep hills and lots of steps are still tiring, but it has improved a lot since I wrote the case study. My feet get very cold easily since then but my arms are as good as before the illness. I have been able to return to work, increasing my hours and changing to a job in a minor injury unit, and I am studying to be an Emergency Nurse Practitioner at university. I have continued to be involved with my children's activities as much as possible, and have helped with many school outings over the years. Best of all I have my friends – I have been able to give something back to my old friends and made lots of new friends, who keep me active and happy.

Janet   DM
59 years old

1994/1995

During a time of huge and protracted stress in the family, (the death of three parents within six months, other long-standing stress related illness in family members) I noticed an itchy rash on my face. I was treated for eczema and dermatitis, and then I found a more fitting description of my symptoms in a medical dictionary. My doctor got me a swift appointment in the dermatology department of the hospital, and I was diagnosed straight away with dermatomyositis. (They were quite impressed that I had found it myself!)

I spent a week in hospital being checked for cancer, (none found) and started on steroids and hydroxychloroquine. I did not get any particular muscle weakness until a year later, when I went into hospital again, this time for three weeks, with the rash, weakness and depression. Azathioprine was added to the medication, with amitriptyline and Prozac for depression.

The hospital team were absolutely super, and took the greatest care of me. I had regular check-ups, I was allowed to discuss my medication and take control of it with their permission. I was made to feel special, which I'm sure had more to do with the rarity of my disease than any personal qualities! But I knew that I could ring my doctor at the hospital at any time, and get a quick appointment if necessary.

1995/2001

During the first few years I felt very sorry for myself and spent a lot of time leaning on my friends and family, my church, and the contacts I made through the Myositis Support Group. I kept working (private tuition) because I had to, and because I love my job! I'm so glad I did keep on, but it was very tough.

I felt there was some improvement when I started the azathioprine tablets, and gradually it seemed that the rash was going. It took four more years, and I could still fall over a blade of grass. (I became terrified of falling, as this was the worst aspect of my weakened legs.)

Then, in 1999 I started on the research trials led by Dr. David Scott, based in Kings College Hospital, London. The exercises, plus the creatine (or placebo, I still don't know which I had) began to make a real difference. After the six months of the trial, I started going to the local gym twice a week. Dr. R and CM had inspired me to go for it and I haven't looked back!

I am fitter now than I was ten years ago, there is no sign of the rash or weakness, and I'm off all medication for dermatomyositis. In fact, when I started to write this article, I almost had to search around in my memory to recall the name of this disease! At one time, it was all I thought about and I couldn't wait to educate the world about it!

To summarise, I feel that azathioprine really worked for me, whereas steroid treatment had little effect and neither did chloroquine for the rash. The depression was treated conventionally, which worked, but actually getting over the disease did more for my mental health than anything, not surprisingly! The support I had from everyone was fantastic; at no time did I feel I was suffering alone. I can see in retrospect that God answered my prayers for healing, though at the time I was in total despair, very scared and thought I might even die.

One of the super spin-offs from the research trials was that my husband, who has M.E., was advised by Dr. R to start exercising in the gym too. (He always came with me to Kings College, and spent the afternoon asleep in a waiting room chair!) Up to that point, the medical advice had been to rest and there was never a hint that he might actually get better. Today, we go to the gym together and he too is fitter than he has been for years, with more energy and fewer infections.

It hasn't been a pleasant experience, but I have learnt things about myself and others, which I may not have learnt otherwise. I have great respect for the hospital medical teams. My hospital experiences were very positive and encouraging.

It was tough for my husband, but he has been my uncomplaining, always there, ever encouraging soul mate throughout the entire illness.

With difficulty I learnt a little patience with myself. I made some new friends with whom I still communicate by letter or the Internet. I have been able to help and support a friend through a similar illness. Perhaps the most satisfying and optimistic feeling I have is that dermatomyositis is something that happened to me in the past. I know theoretically that I am 'in remission', but as far as I am concerned, a revisit is not an option! I would hope that if the worst happened, I would now have the strength and knowledge to face it and beat it – again.

Update

It is now 2005, I'm 63 and I am still fit and well. I suppose I do have certain symptoms which could be left over from dermatomyositis. I have a slight swallowing problem, my cuticles are a bit red and hard and my scalp itches sometimes. Apart from that, nothing. I am still working, which is a great satisfaction to me, since at the beginning I was certain I would have to take early retirement.

I go to the gym, perhaps not quite as regularly as I once did, but there's a reason for this. I now have a new passion in my life. I have discovered line dancing! Two years ago, on holiday in Spain, I tried a few stumbling steps to some fabulous music and I was hooked. I joined a class on my return and two years later I'm now dancing three or four times a week, going to discos and stomps and thoroughly enjoying myself.

I am still in touch with some of my pen pals from ten years ago (those I found through the Myositis Support Group Newsletter) and mostly we share family news, jokes, photos, good times and bad.

In retrospect, though I would never wish to go through the experience again, I can see that dermatomyositis has changed my life for the better, in many ways. I have been one of the lucky ones and I never forget that. I do know that a lot of prayer covered me at the time and gradually I learned to be optimistic as I could see the small but definite improvements which eventually led to my recovery.

Female **DM**
68 years old

I retired from teaching in July 1994 and the following February (95) a rash appeared on my forehead and chest. I was embarrassed at stripping off for my weekly swimming session, so I consulted my GP – a pleasant lady in a large practice.

Firstly, I was put on steroid cream, which did no good and was then referred to the skin consultant at the local hospital. My first meeting with him in June 1995 was traumatic. He told me I had a rare condition – derma-etc of which no one seemed to have heard!!

Within a week I was in hospital for tests – exhaustive and exhausting – blood, urine, blood pressure, x-rays of lungs and breasts, a skin biopsy and finally an electromyogram (very painful) at a neighbouring hospital to which I was taken by taxi!

Then the consultant informed me that I was lucky as only the muscles in my thighs and upper arms were affected by the dermatomyositis!! At this stage I hadn't realised muscles were affected!!

Later that summer I was prescribed prednisolone. This soon helped the large watery blisters, which had formed on my thighs.

My own GP admitted that I was her first case of DM, but the senior partner had had some experience of the condition and took an active interest in my case.

I take Didronel PMO to cut down the risk of osteoporosis and another drug to ward off indigestion etc. At one time I also took another pill to counteract the itch on my skin.

I am now on 5mg prednisolone per day, but I still have the rash –

mainly on my shoulders and lower back. It is very red and itchy (and quite embarrassing!)

I still attend the skin clinic every three months where my consultant is charming – again very sympathetic.

My mother lived until she was 90 and was very healthy most of her life. My father was asthmatic from childhood and died in his early fifties. He suffered from eczema like most asthmatics, so questions were asked of me – whether I had ever had eczema, dermatitis etc – to which the answer was NO!

I have been very active all my life with my teaching, organising school concerts, end of term presentations etc. My main hobby was choral singing and I have sung in thirty consecutive Edinburgh Festivals, made recordings and travelled with the Chorus.

I still ask myself 'Why me?' in respect of my condition – don't we all? Now my muscles don't worry me as much as my skin. I can't take a bath – or rather, I could, but possibly wouldn't get out of the water again as my thigh muscles are still weak, but I have a shower over the bath which is a Godsend!

I enjoy cooking and try to eat wholesome food. I won't say I don't drink! I love France and French cuisine and am sure a glass of wine per day is very beneficial!!

I still suffer from an itchy scalp and flaky fingernails – my consultant says flaky nails are part of our condition!

I try to remain positive about my condition. I have plenty of hobbies – photography, cross-stitch, theatre, opera, ballet and music. I am also a volunteer guide at a local National Trust property.

I have suffered from questions like: -

'Have you been too long in the sun?'

'Have you got nettle rash?'

I then have to go into a long explanation of what DM is!

I'll never forget how isolated I felt when I heard the word 'dermatomyositis' and was told that it was an autoimmune disease.

Update

Alas, I have had a flare up (Nov 2004). My consultant had to put up my dose of prednisolone but I am now gradually tapering again. The rash has appeared again in different places e.g. wrists, outside of both thighs, scalp and the top of both arms (near the shoulder). I am using Betnovate cream during the day and Epaderm ointment on my hands at night to prevent the skin drying.

My consultant says that my DM shouldn't be affected by stress. I think otherwise as my dear friend's condition has worsened and she is now in hospital. I have lost my appetite, am sleeping very badly and have lost a lot of weight. Doesn't that sound like stress??? However, I must feel positive; I visit her daily and have taken over all the driving of our jointly owned car which I might add has been van-dalized twice since Christmas – more stress!!

One good thing I can say is that I have no pain in my muscles just now.

Jane   DM

My story is one of success and may be of inspiration to other sufferers.

My name is Jane and I am married to Fred, my second husband, and have two daughters, Suzanne and Dawn, from my first marriage. Their ages at the time of my illness were thirteen and eleven.

It was January 1989 and Fred's youngest daughter, Ellen, died after a very short illness at the age of twenty-three. We were, of course, all deeply shocked and devastated. Soon after I noticed that I had pins and needles in my hands for an hour or so after waking up each morning. This quickly included swollen knuckles, painful joints and weakness in other joints. Walking up and down stairs, getting in and out of a chair and opening a tin or jar were fast becoming impossible. Suzanne and Dawn had to do little tasks for me before leaving for school each morning.

Every test my doctor did came back negative. We wondered if the shock of Ellen's death had somehow triggered all this off?

March saw my 40th birthday and we decided to go ahead with our planned party as we thought it would be good for the family. My present from Fred was an eternity ring that was several sizes bigger than my wedding and engagement rings, which I could no longer wear. Although I felt quite well on my birthday it wasn't long before my illness really began to take hold.

I was finding some difficulty in swallowing and became breathless very quickly. Every night I would wake in agony with 'dead arms'. My doctor suggested I hung my arm out of the bed, but then it was impossible to move it back in again! Fred said my temperature was very high at night too. Every joint in my body was swollen and painful. My fingers, still swollen, became very sore and dry and the tips were peeling. No cream helped. My fingers felt numb although when anyone touched them they felt hot. Then I thought I had developed an allergy to my eye make-up as my eyelids became puffy and sore too. I kept falling over and became very depressed. The worst thing was not knowing what was wrong with me.

In May I went into hospital for bed rest and tests. At one point they diagnosed me with rheumatoid arthritis, but my consultant wasn't happy with this and arranged one more test which led to the diagnosis of dermatomyositis. I had never heard of it and was frightened by the sound of it. I was put on a high dose of prednisolone and improvement began almost straight away.

Part of my treatment was physiotherapy in the hospital pool and I found I couldn't swim any more; my muscles just wouldn't work! After two years I was off the steroids and back to normal. I do have some weakness in my wrists and sometimes the muscles in my arms hurt, but if I'm careful and rest, it goes. I also get tired more quickly than I used to but otherwise I'm fine.

I now work part time in a small local Boots. Fred and I enjoy walking with our dog in the countryside and on the beach. Sometimes I wonder if I really did have DM as my symptoms, although bad and very disabling at the time, were nowhere near as severe as the ones I read about in the Myositis Support Group newsletter. Perhaps it was just a mild form of the disease. I just know that I am very lucky and thank all the medical staff who helped me to get well and my family and friends for all their support and prayers.

Update

I am still in good health with no recurrence of the symptoms. I don't need to see my consultant anymore, so without tempting providence I would consider myself cured and very lucky!

I do occasionally still get very tired and the muscles in my arms hurt a bit, also my wrists are weak – not helped by breaking my right wrist just over a year ago (which also caused some arthritis to develop in my hand.

I am doing very well.

Jill   DM
57 years old. Diagnosed aged 53

Following a mastectomy I had a silicone implant in July 2001 and then in September of that year I started to feel unwell; hot, fatigued, rapid pulse, high blood pressure and a photosensitive rash. Also I was sore on the nail beds of both hands and very itchy everywhere. My GP referred me to a dermatologist, but I could not wait so I went to our occupational health dept (I work for the NHS) and saw a consultant that same morning. In January 2002 I was diagnosed as having DM, in less than 5 hours! I then commenced hydroxychloroquine, which helped enormously and within weeks I felt better. Initially the rash was where I had caught the sun, so the swim wear mark was clearly evident, then it was the knuckles, nail beds and later the pink eyelids, but they have all subsided.

As the summer months progressed I improved and gradually discontinued the medication. When the winter (2002-2003) commenced I had a flare up so I recommenced the medication. The following summer I improved again and took myself off the medication. I started swimming and can now swim up to a mile at a session and that has helped. Last winter and this winter I have not needed to take any medication. I discovered florescent lighting triggers the DM. However, I am able to manage this.

I discharged myself from the consultant feeling empowered, after having read the first edition of this book and attending two myositis conferences.

I became a participant in one of the expert patient programmes at the end of last year. I then went on a course in January 2005 and am now a volunteer tutor with the group. This has enabled me to further learn how to manage the DM by learning to meditate etc.

www.expertpatients.nhs.uk

Expert patients are people living with a long-term health condition who are able to take more control over their health by understanding and managing their conditions, leading to an improved quality of life.

Some of the benefits are:

* Feel confident and in control of their lives
* Aim to manage their condition and its treatment in partnership with health care professionals
* Communicate effectively with professionals and are willing to share responsibility on treatment
* Are realistic about the impact of their disease on themselves and their family
* Use their skills and knowledge to lead full lives.

I recently had a total hip replacement. Being in hospital, the florescent lights and the surgery, affected my DM and I felt recovery took a bit longer than normal. But to date I feel very well and much of my fitness has returned. I go swimming and walking which both help the DM. I also work 30 hours a week

The only drug I ever took was hydroxychloroquine and the occasional Ibuprofen.

My CPK levels were always within normal range. However, I did feel as though I was walking through treacle at times. My thighs felt very 'heavy' and I often felt I could not take another step. Also, I used to and still get, to a slighter degree, joint pains, but they do not affect the daily activities of living.

I am now returning to my previous fitness level, although I do get fatigued and the DM does flare up (pink all over and aching especially in my legs and more recently my neck) However, I have DM and it hasn't got me!

Maureen   **DM/PM**
46 years old. Diagnosed aged 19

I am not sure where to begin. I am 46 years old, female and living in Sydney Australia. I am from Scotland and first had polymyositis when I was 19 and living in Scotland. I was very ill at that time and spent 6 months in a Glasgow hospital. I don't remember everything about that time but had real difficulty with just about everything: sitting up, walking, talking, had no swallow for about 4 weeks and was fed by a tube.

I had lots of steroids which didn't seem to help and then plasma phere-sis. That seemed to make the difference for me. I reduced the steroids very slowly over two years and regained all my muscle strength.

I left Scotland for Australia in 1980. The funny thing was no one ever told me I had a disease! I just thought I had a strange illness that had gone away and that was the end of it. I had no check ups or drugs for the next 23 years! I never even thought about my past illness. I got married, had 3 kids, went to work every day and had a normal life.

Out of the blue, about the middle of 2002, I started with a red eye-lid; it got worse over a few weeks and the doctor thought I had an aller-gy. Then the other eyelid got red and I had a rash on my arms. The doctor then sent me to a skin specialist. I mentioned to her that I had had polymyositis years ago. She examined me and found I also had the rash on my chest, back and fingers. She said she was very sorry, but she was sure I had dermatomyositis. She took a skin biopsy to confirm this. She got me an urgent appointment with a rheumatologist and gave me a discount on my bill as she was so sorry to give me this bad news! It was all down hill after that muscle biopsy in December, then on to high dose steroids the next day. It was getting worse by the day!

The week between Christmas and New Year I just lay in bed and watched my arms and legs melt away to nothing. I lost 10kg that week and knew I was in trouble. I started to have swallowing trouble again and that really scared me. My doctor was away on holiday and I had his mobile number but didn't feel right about calling him. By New Year's Eve I had to go to hospital and of course they had to admit me. They started me off on the pulse of steroids (3 lots of steroids by IV). This made no difference at all. They gave me IV Immunoglobulin for 5 days and my swallowing started to improve and I wanted to go home. I went home still very weak and unable to look after myself. I was on very high dose prednisone, methotrexate and calcium and folic acid etc.

I went into hospital every month until August for IVIG and managed to reduce the steroids over the months. I am now on a low dose of steroids and the methotrexate. I am back to being able to look after myself and the family with no real weakness, but I do get very tired by afternoon and forget the evenings!

I hope to return to work next month for 2 days per week. I work at a school so I am lucky to have lots of holidays.

I should add that I am one of these people who have never had a very high CK and in fact it has never been more than 600. It has remained around 30 for a few months.

Vidhi   DM
29 years old. Diagnosed aged 20

This is a story of a girl to whom muscles were the most important aspect of her body. She was a qualified aerobic instructor and a personal trainer teaching almost five classes a day. She was studying Sports Medicine at the University of Charleston, USA with a dream to open a fitness club and attain the Master Trainer title when she graduated. She is now a full time merchandiser with Marks & Spencer with a job that is primarily desk based. She has dermatomyositis. This girl is me.

This is how my story goes … in the summer of 96, I was back home in India on my summer holiday. My sisters and I decided to take a trip up to the Greater Himalayas, abode of gods and visit the valley of flowers. It was a 700km's drive, which takes almost two nights and two days one way and I was determined to come back in five days, as I had to attend to my students. We reached Badrinath where we had booked ourselves in a hotel with views overlooking another peak. While we sat sipping our morning tea, my younger sister proposed we climb the peak we could see from our balcony. Our aim was to reach the glacier from where the river Ganges originates. Since I was an aerobic instructor, the goal did not seem a problem at all. Little did I know what was in store for me when I started the climb. So we city girls, with hardly any trekking equipment and wearing our jeans and trainers, took off to climb. As we were hiking, I was taking short breaks after every few minutes and since I was the only fitness instructor of the whole group, I had to keep up my reputation. They all talked about how serene the mountains were making them feel. But internally, my body was far from serene. I felt that there was a volcano about to erupt. After a lot effort from my side, we finally reached the peak. I have to say, it was worth the effort. The mountains were absolutely magnificent and the beauty of the place temporarily made me forget how I was feeling.

We came back after few days and I noticed that I had two little rashes on my forehead. I did not make anything out of it and decided that it was probably sunburn from the mountains. Even when I was teaching my classes, it was a lot of effort to conduct them. I would teach the sequence and then had to make the excuse of walking around to check the students, whilst, in fact, I was unable to cope with the sequence myself. I was feeling a lot of pain in my joints, especially the knees and knuckles. I showed myself to a general practitioner in India and he referred me to an orthopaedic doctor. That day when I saw the consultant, I was mortified. After having some blood tests done, his prognosis was rheumatoid arthritis even though the RF factor came out to be negative. He explained the condition to me in such dramatic manner. He said that my fingers would go all twisted and I would have trouble pickings things up. He then gave me some exercises for the fingers. On top of these exercises, he prescribed a malaria tablet, which seems to treat Arthritis. I was still determined to go back to the US and finish my semester. So, I went back.

It was in America that my real DM symptoms started. My gums started to bleed and I had severe mouth ulcers. Anything I ate had to be completely bland with no spices and cold. Trust me, when you are in a university you really do not have much choice with food. So I ended up eating nothing at all. I was just living on cucumbers and tomatoes. As the days went by, my condition was getting worse and worse. I was starting to have trouble climbing stairs, washing my hair and even picking things up from the floor. I kept pushing myself as I had assignments to do, classes to attend and on top of that I was also teaching my aerobic classes to earn some pocket money for the week. Then the butterfly rash appeared on my face and also rashes on my knuckles. I looked so ugly and could not bear to look at my face in the mirror. My hair started to fall out and I started losing a lot of weight. Obviously, more and more often, I was calling in sick at the gym and so I lost my aerobic class to another instructor who could actually come and conduct them. There was one time when I woke up one morning and I could not get up. I had absolutely no strength to lift myself up to even go to the bathroom. That was the day I realized that something was really seriously wrong with me. I somehow managed to call India and speak to my father who sent my sister to fetch me and get me back home. I left my course half way through and went back to India.

All this time, I still thought that I had rheumatoid arthritis but the tablets were not benefiting me. Every single morning my mother had to physically pick me up in order to feed me some breakfast. The food would give me some energy and I would just about manage to get up and have a shower. Bed had become my favourite place and TV my best friend. And then, by some fate, my brother-in law uncle came visiting from the US. He was a rheumatologist at the Mayo Clinic, Washington. I went to see him for a second opinion. He looked at my face, checked my fingers and pretty much knew what I had. But he reserved his judgment until he got some blood tests done. He instructed me to have my CK level tested. Low and behold, it came back high and he diagnosed me with dermatomyositis. No one had ever heard of this condition in India. We managed to find a local rheumatologist who had studied about it but had never treated this condition. He prescribed 60 mg of prednisolone, methotrexate and some tummy medications to counteract the steroids. I took this medication for almost 6 months and started to see some relief. My condition started to settle down and my routine became somewhat normal. Although as anyone taking methotrexate will probably know, it does have a negative effect on the body. I lost even more hair and on the days I took it, I pretty much stayed in bed since it made me feel incredibly drowsy. But on the whole, I was getting better.

Eventually, after taking this medication for a good year, I started to taper the steroids. As, I was getting my energy back, I felt that I was getting cured and decided to completely stop taking any medication. I was actually fine, living a normal life and even had started to personally train one client for almost a year. And then, I met my husband who had come on holiday to India for a week. Low and behold, we fell in love and got married and I came to the UK. I was still not taking any medication and thought that I had been cured. But, it was not to be. After a year in the UK, I came down with a flare. I spoke to Jenny, who has become my very close friend. She referred me to her consultant and he yet again diagnosed my flare as relapse of DM. Back on steroids and on methotrexate.

However, this time around I have taken it very carefully. I am still on medication but on a very low dose of steroids. I am working full time at Marks & Spencer as a merchandiser. I regularly swim and exercise and have also registered to attend a yoga teacher training course that starts soon. Touch wood, I am living as fit a life as I possibly can. There is a lot of control and discipline required as my body has limited energy and I have to use that energy in the most effective way. It is hard sometimes, as in corporate world you are required to work long hours and maintain networks; I am required to go out in the evening for drinks occasionally. Late nights and alcohol really tire me out and wipe me out completely the following day. I have to find a fine balance between my work, socializing, maintaining a house and marriage and fitness. But, one saving grace is that my husband is a real superstar. He helps me a lot in the house and cooks me dinner when I have had a very long day.

I am lucky, because I have a life-support system built of friends and family, who are both sensitive to and supportive of my condition. Especially my husband, who makes the best mash in the world, my sisters and parents who have seen me come out of this damn illness and have boosted my confidence in those no hair days and Jenny, who is always there whenever I need her and who actually understands what it is to have DM. I urge all those who endure the vicissitudes of myositis to find or even start a similar support group – because they are there and those who are available, without condition, who will help to see you through the hard times. Never feel you are alone.

To end this article, all I can say to all those people with any type of myositis is that the brain is stronger than the body. We all need to listen to our bodies; for example, I listened to mine and yoga called. It works for me and I shall soon be teaching a class in restorative yoga (you are all invited to attend). The key is to fight DM; it is not a battle; it is a war – which all sufferers can win. We can fight it. And so we should fight it. We CAN.

Case Studies – Polymyositis

Pauline   **PM**
52 years old. Diagnosed aged 45.

I was diagnosed with primary Sjogrens syndrome and secondary polymyositis in 1995. This was after a considerable amount of time spent doing the rounds of various hospitals.

Looking back, I realize I had not been well for about 2 years prior to that. I eventually went to the doctor because I had a recurrent rash on my legs, which I had put down to an allergy! I tried everything from changing my soap, detergent, wearing cotton all the time, tried various creams etc. all to no avail. Eventually one day the rash was so bad that it frightened me. This is crazy I thought, I really ought to go to see my GP. So along I went and apologized most profusely for bothering the doctor over such a trivial thing.

He got me a bit worried as he ordered some blood tests (what on earth do I need blood tests for when I've only got a rash I thought). Later that week my own doctor rang and said I should go back for some more blood tests as my blood was showing some abnormalities. It so happened that I had managed to catch a virus the day after going to the doctor so I thought the abnormalities must be due to this (I was innocent in those days!)

The second set of blood tests sent me off in a hurry to see a haematologist – gosh I've got leukemia I thought! Yet more blood tests and I was very bluntly told that I had got rheumatoid arthritis and I'd also got a nuclear factor in my blood – any minute now I'm going to explode I thought!

I didn't have an ache in any of my joints so how could I possibly have rheumatoid arthritis? So off to a rheumatologist it was, who, yes, you've guessed it, ordered more blood tests and as the results slowly filtered through I had more and more blood tests – it seems my blood is most peculiar! Still no symptoms to speak of so it was next off to a meeting of rheumatologists where I was one of their 'interesting' cases – there were about 50 specialists at this meeting which was a bit scary! They came to no conclusion either.

However, later on I started to feel my legs were getting a bit weaker (I've also had polio) so my rheumatologist thought it might be a good idea to have some physiotherapy. One day I went back to be checked and the physiotherapist was very cross with me because she was convinced that I had been sitting on my backside doing nothing – but I hadn't – I had been doing everything I normally do, plus all the exercises. When I eventually managed to persuade her that I was telling the truth she immediately referred me back to my rheumatologist who then decided he wanted a biopsy of my eyelid (not sure of the medical reasons for this one!) Then it was an EMG and a muscle biopsy. Lo and behold a diagnosis was made – and all of it due to a physiotherapist!

A massive 'bomb' of steroids, then a visit to see Professor I. who is responsible for dictating my treatment but my care is overseen locally. Steroids were a miracle worker for me. I gradually taper the steroids and add methotrexate into the pot. A Dexa scan to check for osteoporosis and then HRT and calcium supplements are added into the pot! Hopefully that will keep my bones strong and healthy!

I'm now relatively healthy although I have lost some muscle power in my legs (running is impossible) and I am unable to walk long distances and also walk a lot slower than I used to. I'm down to 5mg steroids and 7.5mg methotrexate and I'm still trying to taper even further. I am one of the lucky ones who never put on any weight when on high dose steroids.

Having this disease has made me a lot more sympathetic and understanding to people who have physical difficulties. I have also had minor adjustments made to our house – like adding a second banister, taps that are easy to turn on and a new kitchen with easy access cupboards etc. Next on the list is an extra handrail for the bath. I know I'm fortunate because I can carry on working, as I'm in a job where I can sit down for most of the day.

On medical advice I was told to adopt a low fat, no red meat diet. I do eat lamb still but have cut out beef entirely. I do believe this has helped. I also take cod liver oil and oil of evening primrose.

I have taken part in a 'Creatine supplementation' trial (results await-ed). This involved doing about 20 minutes of exercise a day as well as taking Creatine or the placebo! I found these exercises very helpful and firmly believe that everyone with this disease should be encour-aged to exercise as best they can. I think it would be a good idea if an exercise video was made for people with mild/moderate myositis and also moderate/severe myositis. With any luck, a physiotherapist read-ing this will take up this idea!

I also feel it is important to remain positive. OK, so I can no longer run after the men, (which is a bit disastrous at my age!) but I can and do have a lot more time to listen to people. I read more than I used to and have just recently started gardening again (light tasks only). I also play the flute in my spare time. In the early days of the disease I could not manage to play for very long and withdrew from public perfor-mances and teaching, but recently I played in a concert (yes, I was tired at the end of it – but I did it!)

My message to anyone suffering from this disease is keep positive. You will have bad days but you will also have good days. Keep active and keep mixing with other people. Join the Myositis Support Group and try to learn as much about the disease as possible. Eat a good, bal-anced, low fat diet and that includes at least five pieces of fruit or veg-etables and remember the old proverb 'USE IT OR LOSE IT!'

Update

I remain much the same as I was with the possible exception that my thigh muscles have got weaker, which means going up and down stairs is beginning to become a bit of a problem. I also had great fun trying to get out of a boat recently!

I had my first major flare up, since diagnosis, just before Christmas 2004 and had to have my drugs increased, but things are beginning to settle again and I am now back on my bike. I have just started training to be a CAB adviser and I help run a Babe and Toddler Group for my church so I am keeping quite active. I also play the flute and I have formed a small flute group. We play at old peo-

ple's homes etc. I have a dog that I try to walk regularly, albeit slowly! The reason for me telling you this, is that there is life after myositis. Don't let it beat you. You may not be able to do so much physical activity but you can do other things instead. As an example, we have various working parties at our church; gardening, painting etc. I am not able to take part in these, but I can help make the teas and I can help with the paperwork etc. so I feel I'm doing my bit. Most of all try to keep cheerful and take an active interest in other people – it helps to keep your mind off your own problems.

I took part in the Creatine Trial at Kings College and I have recently been told I was on the placebo. Whilst I was doing the trial I was given a number of exercises to do every day (or at least every other day), in addition to this you had to try to walk or cycle for 20 minutes each day. At the end of the trial, I did feel that I was more confident in walking and that I had improved very slightly. I was not surprised when I was told that I was on the placebo, and it was good to hear that those people who were on the Creatine did make slightly better progress than those on the placebo – so it may be worth trying Creatine if you haven't already done so.

Susan   **PM**

At the age of 15 I had glandular fever and never felt quite right after that. Years followed fairly normally until 25 when I had a stomach virus, it took me over nine months to recover. The hospital just said it would take time. I returned to work but stomach bugs kept pulling me down. At 28 I collapsed several times and was sent home from work, unable to walk properly, exhausted, dizzy with nausea and having trouble with my speech. I saw my doctor and unfortunately mentioned I was vegan (bad move!) He said I was malnourished with low blood sugar and told me to eat meat and plenty of sugar. I returned to living but passed out again. I knew there was something seriously wrong and went for a second opinion. This new doctor diagnosed me with ME. I went to see various specialists who then started to say 'but you don't normally have those symptoms with ME.' I then saw a specialist who said I had been diagnosed with ME at my last hospital visit when I was 25! Two years of tests led to a muscle biopsy that concluded that I had polymyositis.

A change of diet helped, kept vegan, but simple, plain and softer so I could swallow and digest it more easily. Also an anti-candida diet. My partner was an ex weight lifter and managed to find in the muscle builder supplements, a soya protein which I added to my meal when it was a 'not eating properly time'. Once I reached a certain stage, I felt I had to exercise. I started once a day to try to walk around the small raised shrubs in the garden. A bit like the 1962 film 'Twice round the daffodils.' When I reached 25 rounds I then attempted my first walk outside the house in years. I now exercise regularly. I also went to see a Reiki healer who helped enormously. I set myself targets each day, so I had a reason to get up, no matter how small, just so that I could achieve something. When I started to improve, I attempted home study courses to give me focus.

My parents and my partner Ian were my main supporters to help me cope. Mum and Dad gave me a safe home and constant care. Ian was always at the end of a phone and guided me in an exercise programme to help me gain mobility. My stubborn independent character and my desire to return to work helped me to fight PM.

I thought I wanted to die because I had lost everything dear to me, but a profound experience changed that. This is what brings me to the positive side of my illness…

I was scared to be left alone. I didn't want to die alone. On many nights when I went to sleep, I would start to drift down a dark tunnel and feel I was leaving my body. I had to fight the pull and I kept repeating I don't want to leave.

Yet the darkness was taking me somewhere good – I could feel that – but I didn't want to give up so soon on my life – there were things I wanted to do. I never believed in life after death or a spirit life but now I do. I've also met others who have shared their spiritual experiences and it's fascinated me. I lean towards no particular religion. I could never allow myself restrictions after what I've been through, but whatever I do, I try to do it for the good. I have been given a second chance to stay and I hope to get things right. I now know I do not wish to die yet, but I was just tired of the nothingness that severe illness makes you feel.

I had never considered alternative medicine, until main stream medicine had given up on me. But it has opened up a whole new world! I'm into crystals, herbs and different forms of healing – the list is vast! I've changed my direction in life now. I used to be a party animal living on the surface.

Ian and I had only been together a year before I became ill and it made me realize that he genuinely cared.

I see people completely differently now. I thought I had to be surrounded by them to survive, but I'm not that important to anyone. They are a bonus to my life, not a reason for my existence. I've learnt that I am stronger than I realized and have become a more independent thinker, not seeking approval any more. I think I am more honest too, life is too short to pretend. I've proved people wrong, a triumphant feeling. One doctor told me that I would never work again. I am – part-time, but I'm doing it! I am also developing my own business to give me total control of my working life. This has led me to appear in our local newspaper. I always wanted to be famous! I now know I just want to be well and happy – so I'm working on both! In my business I am trying to give people the HOPE that I never had. By doing that, it is helping me. People I meet now say I am very positive and very sure of what I want, yet most of them don't know I've had years of isolation to sit and contemplate. That is a definite advantage of having myositis – MAGICAL MIND MOMENTS!

I have the courage to work towards things, because I feel I have lost out on so much. I don't want to miss out on anything else!

I do have a tendency to push myself too far and my body soon reminds me and I'm sure it always will, but what I have now is far beyond what I thought I would ever be doing. To walk down my road and get on a bus is a sheer delight. One of many things most people take for granted and which I will always be reminded never to do. I've written myself letters and short descriptions at different stages of my illness, that are there to read to remind me that it has been worse. I am drawn to people with disabilities. I know I was looked at and spoken to as if I was abnormal by well people. Inside my head I knew I was just the same as them, and they had no right to make me feel less than I was. I want people to feel good about themselves and now I try my best to help people find that. Myositis has helped me experience a piece of the heavy side of life that most people would not glimpse. I hope they never do. I have no regrets because of the knowledge I have gained.

I asked my partner Ian, what he thought was a positive aspect of my illness, he said the following:

'The only positive aspect that I see about Susan having Myositis is that she has found out who her true friends are.'

Update

I have not improved in the last two years and having collapsed several times it has been harder to return from each set back. Yet, there has been more in my life to deal with, so it is no surprise. I have managed to keep my part-time job, but it has been a struggle! The mind is willing whilst the body does not quite agree!

My resolve still stands to take one day at a time and make the best of what I have. I try not to plan or think of the future. That way I avoid disappointment!

This doesn't mean I have no hope, but to set unrealistic targets is not positive planning. Simplicity is super, sensational and most of all achieveable. These are the joys that lead to the seeds of success.

Chris (Female)   PM/Overlap
52 years old

This is the story of my diagnosis of polymyositis and how I have coped so far.

After feeling unwell and a little weak in March 2000, I started getting red ring like rashes on the tops of my arms.

After going to the doctors' several times and given different creams for a fungal infection, I was referred to the dermatology clinic at our local hospital, where a biopsy and blood tests were taken. After a few months they came to the conclusion that I had subacute lupus.

I then noticed my legs getting weak and climbing the stairs became like climbing a mountain. I was in between appointments at the clinic and started to read medical books! On discovering DM/PM and the symptoms, I was convinced that this was what I had and it did not make for very good reading. I was very frightened at some of the things that I read.

When I went for my next appointment I told the doctor about my weakness and suggested that I may have this very rare disease. She agreed to do more tests and a fortnight later I was told that this was in fact what I had! That week I was taken into hospital and stayed for two and a half weeks where I had lots of different tests to see if I had cancer along with this disease.

Just before I went into hospital I felt at my lowest ebb and I think I hit rock bottom mentally. I was in total despair.

Once in hospital, I felt I was getting to grips with it and happy that at last things were being done. I left hospital and was told that everything seemed clear apart from enlarged lymph nodes on my liver, which they believed was due to the myositis.

However, armed with all the drugs and steroids I have gradually got myself back to normality, almost anyway! I feel so much better and stronger taking the steroids and just want to say that in those dark, dark days, I never thought I would bounce back as well as I have.

I know that I have to live with the disease, but things now don't seem so bleak as when I first became aware of this disease. Speaking with fellow sufferers (not many of us) helps a great deal and I now feel less isolated and much more positive about life and the future.

Update

First the positive. I am still able to get around and I am glad I am not in too much pain. Unfortunately, I still take lots of pills. Four months ago they had to put my prednisolone up as I had a flare when I got below 7.5 mg per day. I am also on methotrexate.

Two years ago I was diagnosed with Type 2 diabetes which I am convinced is due to the steroids and now I have to take metformin for this. I have also developed osteoarthritis of the knee which is painful and quite debilitating but I have learnt to live with it. I have had high blood pressure for many years but this has increased since having myositis and being on steroids. However, I am grateful that I can still get around but like to have my husband around so that I can hang onto his arm. The hardest thing to contend with at the moment is the fatigue. I have good days and bad days, when I could sleep all day. I live very near the main hospital for us and see my consultant every 2-3 months. I try to keep upbeat most of the time and, as I said, I am glad I am not in severe pain.

Hillary   **PM**
59 years old

In July 1999 I was diagnosed as suffering from rheumatoid arthritis. I had a constant temperature of 100+, joint pain and limitation, general feeling of lethargy and depression. I was treated with gold injections, methotrexate, Arthrotec and sulphasalazine. I later changed from Arthrotec to naproxen. I already took thyroxine for an underactive thyroid gland.

Mid August 2001 I started some different symptoms to the RA; heavy muscles, exhaustion, permanent temperature, lethargy, no appetite, breathlessness. As these symptoms increased, so the RA became less obvious. By September I was unable to cross my legs or lift them into the car without manually doing so with my hands. Mid October I was signed off work as I could hardly do anything for myself and 13 November was admitted to hospital. CK levels read 9,000. By that time I had less than 10% muscle power and was unable to swallow at all. I spent eight weeks in hospital and then had a 'peg' directly into my stomach. The 'peg' was removed in April 2001 once I was becoming self sufficient with swallowing.

The diagnosis was polymyositis coupled with vasculitis. I was given Cyclophosphamide chemotherapy, immunoglobulin and hydrocortisone. I had been on 60mg daily of prednisolone before I went into hospital and this dropped to 20 mg daily as the chemo was ongoing. Fortunately I did not lose my hair but it went very thin. In the middle of all this I suffered a DVT and as I have had pulmonary emboli twice in the past, will have to be on warfarin permanently. I left hospital mid January 2001.

During the next few months I was taking thyroxine and warfarin and the prednisolone dosage gradually came down to 10mg daily but the CK levels went up to 6,000 again and I went back into hospital again in September 2001 to start another course of chemo/immunoglobulin and hydrocortisone.

I had been doing quite well but again, the prednisolone came down too low and my CK levels are now up to 2,900 so I am back on 40mg daily. Obviously I am still on thyroxine and now take hydroxychloroquine sulphate and warfarin.

Apart from the drug regime, there seems to be no rhyme nor reason for taking a sudden dip and feeling dreadful. On 3rd January 2002, my husband had a heart attack and is now suffering from angina. Just as he hoped to go back to work part-time early April, he was made redundant. Probably both our health situations affect the other, stress wise.

July 2002 saw another week in hospital for five days of immunoglobulin, reduction in prednisolone to 30 and then 20mg daily. Methotrexate has been reintroduced, now up to 15mg weekly, folic acid 5mg 6 days per week and hydroxychloroquine sulphate stopped.

Throughout the whole saga, my husband, children, friends and colleagues have been very supportive. My son, who is a Coeliac, found the whole business very difficult to cope with, especially the 'peg'. My grandchildren were upset, but made me lots of get well cards and we spoke on the phone a lot. They asked lots of questions which I tried to answer as honestly as possible.

I have been so fortunate that my consultant and the ward staff at my hospital have supported my husband and me in every way possible. The medical team have been open and honest with us. The consultant is happy to discuss our concerns and there is mutual trust in the relationships. There is no doubt this support has been instrumental in helping us come to terms with what has happened.

The effects of the drugs were nearly as bad as the condition. The large doses of steroids made me extremely agitated and aggressive and unable to sleep – my poor husband went to hell and back! I have also put on weight and although it starts to drop as the steroid dosage comes down, the weight rockets as soon as the dosage is lifted. This depresses me more than anything. Apart from pregnancy, I have always been a size 10 but now a 14.

I have had to take ill-health retirement from a job I loved. I was an H R Officer for a large crop protection company and was fortunate to have every possible support from them. This has been a big hurdle to cross, coming to terms with losing my job/independence.

Update

The last time I had immunoglobin treatment was May/June 2002 when, for no apparent reason my CK soared to 3500. Since then my body seems to have reached a tolerance level and my CK levels hover between 30 and 50. There have been minor 'flare ups' and bed rest /

medication increases have been necessary. The swallowing problem occasionally gives me grief (particularly when I get tired) and the aches are as if I have 'flu'. Climbing stairs / steps is difficult.

My medication still includes weekly methotrexate but I am now down to a low dose of prednisolone which has really pleased me although it has been a battle to get there. I do have more joint and muscle pain now, though I am determined not to increase the dosage unless the discomfort gets out of hand or I have big 'flare up'.

In July 2004 my consultant and I decided, as I had been stable for a while, we would try physiotherapy and see how my muscles reacted. We timed it well and I now do a gentle exercise programme for 35mins on alternate days. This has a holistic effect – I feel I am helping myself rather than relying on medication and I have lost weight. The weight issue has always concerned me, both from the health and vanity views!!

Supporting others newly diagnosed has made me feel this saga has not been for nothing and when I hear how others are coping/not coping I realise I am very fortunate to have come this far.

Freda   **PM**
57 years old

I was diagnosed with polymyositis and connective tissue disease just over six years ago, when I was 50 years old.

I had had a year of repeated visits to doctors, being told, 'I was depressed. It was my age'. etc. etc.) When I reached the stage of not being able to walk or swallow I was referred to a consultant at our local hospital. After a brief examination and some blood tests I was sent away with these words, 'Try not to dwell on things, it's possibly your age, and if you can't swallow just think of the weight you can loose'. (I was just under 9st at the time.) 'Just treat yourself to a nice bottle of mineral water that will help you swallow'. I left in tears thinking I was going mad.

Later, the same day, I received a phone call from the same consultant with the news that 'Your blood tests revealed some worrying symptoms'. I was finally admitted to hospital and from then on my life changed.

High doses of steroids caused massive weight gain. I had to give up work. I didn't want to go out anywhere. My family and friends were very supportive but there were days when I didn't want to get out of bed.

Then, just over a year ago a friend persuaded me to go with her to a craft class. Not being a crafty person at first I was reluctant, but I gave it a try. Everyone was very friendly and I was shown how to do 'Pergamano' making greeting cards with parchment paper. It now helps me relax and I have had a lot of pleasure making birthday and Christmas cards for my family and friends. I can't thank my friend, June, enough for persuading me to go with her. Although I still have problems, I have found a talent I would never have known about had I still have been working.

Update

I was diagnosed with PM nine years ago. In that time many combinations of drugs have been tried. At the moment I am on methotrexate and prednisolone but my symptoms have persisted. Recently I was transferred to a different specialist who seemed to think my symptoms related more to IBM and not PM as originally thought. However, after having another muscle biopsy the original diagnosis of PM is correct, so I will have to carry on with the same treatment. They are still unable to tell if the problems I have walking, climbing stairs etc are permanent damage due to the myositis or the steroids weakening the muscle.

As always with this illness weakness is the main problem so lots of activities are limited. Nevertheless, I go to a craft class and spend a lot of time making cards for family and friends. My son has recently given me a computer so I am also spending time trying to remember all of his instructions, often failing miserably!

Jean   **PM**
82 years old. Diagnosed aged 70.

In 1991 I had pain in my limbs, I was 71 and was unable to lift my arms to play bowls, a game I very much enjoyed. I cried a lot with the pain, the worst I had had since labour pains and not over as quickly!

I went to my doctor and he thought it was rheumatism and gave me a series of painkillers. I had masses of these different painkillers, all to no avail.

Myositis was unknown here in Norfolk and still is, on the whole. I asked for a second opinion and my doctor sent me to a rheumatologist. I went as a private patient and as a result of a blood test was admitted to hospital the next day. I had lots of blood tests, nerve conduction electromyography, a muscle biopsy, endoscopy and x-ray. After 4 days I was home again and on steroids and azathioprine.

In June 1991 my CPK reading was 1117 and is now between 30-40 but with several ups and downs over the years.

I am still on steroids, 4mg per day and 50mg azathioprine, obviously a much lower dose now and my consultant says the myositis is inactive, but I do get pain in my legs if I walk far or stand for too long. I rest when I can during the day. I think there are only one or two other cases of myositis at my surgery. I have mild osteoporosis as a result of being on steroids a long time, but that is under control with Fosamax and Calcichew tablets. I also have mild Raynaud's, which is a side effect of myositis and which only affects me in the cold weather when my hands and feet change colour. Apart from all this I keep going with an active brain and a sense of humour.

Update

I must say the illness has progressed and my arms and legs ache a lot. I see my rheumatologist every six months and am still on steroids plus various heart pills. The fact that I am 84 years old does not help. I am very unsteady and now have a stair lift which is a great help as we live upstairs and sleep downstairs. We have a beautiful view over the golf course, beach and sea.

I must say I am struggling but keep going and have what help I can. My husband now has a pacemaker and trouble with his memory since the operation. Never mind, we get by with the help of our daughter who lives locally.

Sadly Jean passed away in December 2005. She was 85 years old. I thank her son for allowing me to publish her case study and update.

Margaret   **PM**
52 years old

My story begins around Christmas 1995. I started experiencing discomfort in my hands. I'm a keen knitter and it hurt to hold the needles. Also I was cycling to work and my hands were uncomfortable holding the handlebars. The discomfort soon spread to my legs and they just didn't feel right!

I visited my GP on several occasions and tried to explain that my body just didn't feel as it should. He carried out neurological tests but couldn't find any problems. He also sent me for x-rays on my hands and a blood test. Nothing unusual showed up. The weakness continued and I had to stop knitting and cycling. My doctor treated me for depression because the situation was getting me down and I was tearful quite often. He also thought my symptoms were psychosomatic! This annoyed me somewhat because I felt that he was not taking me seriously.

By the end of April beginning of May 1996 I felt so debilitated. My ankles and legs were quite swollen and I was signed off work. I could not straighten up if I bent over. I needed help to get off the toilet and had to sit high in an armchair to be able to get up. The stairs became a nightmare because it hurt my legs to climb them and I had to stop taking baths as I did not feel safe and couldn't lift my legs over the side. If I went out I was very unsure on my feet and fell a few times. One time I could not get up again without help. After a while my doctor did refer me to a rheumatologist on the NHS but the appointment was a long time coming through.

In the meantime I consulted another doctor in the practice for a second opinion and asked to be referred through my BUPA insurance. A second blood test showed some abnormalities! At the end of May I saw Dr B, at a Hampshire hospital, who immediately diagnosed polymyositis and admitted me for intensive drug therapy and physiotherapy. I also had a small piece of muscle removed from my right thigh and an electromyogram to confirm the diagnosis. I responded very well to treatment and the relief of getting a firm diagnosis was wonderful because I had been so frightened of what might be wrong with me. I'd had visions of being confined to a wheelchair for the rest of my life. Indeed my son had been pushing me around in one prior to going in hospital! My stay in hospital lasted two and a half weeks and I was off work for a couple of months. There have been a couple of hiccups with my regular blood tests since, but on the whole I feel well and the prednisolone and azathioprine, that I take every day, seem to keep things under control. I continue to work full time and cycle every day.

Until I was diagnosed with PM my friends, my family and I had never heard of PM which apparently is not unusual! They were all very supportive throughout my problems and continue to be so. Particularly my son Matthew.

When I first started taking the steroids I was on quite a large dose and my face became quite puffy which I didn't feel happy with, but as the dose was gradually reduced my face went back to normal. I have gained a couple of stones in body weight over the past six years but I do not entirely blame the medication because I'm also going through the menopause and am a bit of a foodie!

At the time of writing this story I have recently reduced my prednisolone by 1mg a day and I've been getting tingling and burning sensations in my hands, which I have experienced in the past when reducing the steroid dose. Hopefully this will not mean having to increase again.I will not know until I next meet with the specialist. It is my wish that eventually I will be in remission and off all medication as I'm sure is the wish of all sufferers! I try to stay positive about the future and would like to say to anyone who has recently been diagnosed with this nasty condition that there is light at the end of the tunnel!

Best wishes to all of you wherever you are.

Update

Since my original account of how PM affected my life I am pleased to report that my condition is in remission and I'm not taking any medication. The journey from diagnosis to a clean bill of health has taken eight years 1996-2004. I've been advised by the consultant to have my blood tested once every year until further notice and that's it!

I consider myself one of the lucky people because my body

responded well to the treatment of steroids and immunosuppressants and apart from gaining a bit of weight (which I've since lost) I suffered no side effects! In my experience I found acceptance of my condition and living with it and not letting it rule my life helped me to recover and move forward. I tried not to dwell on it. I tried to be positive and stay active by cycling to work every day, walking and taking part in any form of exercise I enjoyed and could manage.

In the same year that I was diagnosed, I took a trip to New York and then a couple of years later I had a holiday in Cyprus. This was followed by a trip to the Far East, which was my dream holiday and one I hope to repeat.

I hope many others have been and will be as successful as I was with their treatment.

Eleanor   PM
52 years old

My story began in 1994, when I was 44, although it probably began a long time before that; fingers turning white in my teens (Raynaud's disease?), burning pains in my thighs, whenever a walk included a steep climb in my twenties. Many allergic type rashes for as long as I can remember.

The pains that started, eight years ago, began in the base of my thumbs and within a couple of months were in all my fingers. The pain was excruciating as my fingers swelled and my nerves were being squeezed. I went to my GP, who took a blood sample and said there was no rheumatoid factor, prescribed ibuprofen and refused to refer me to a specialist. I found a more sympathetic GP, who referred me privately to a rheumatologist, who looked at my by now, swollen knees, ankles and fingers and pronounced it was definitely rheumatoid arthritis.

I then spent the next three years as an outpatient at the rheumatology clinic at a London hospital and was prescribed steroids and Salazopyrin. They acknowledged that you could still have RA without the rheumatoid factor appearing in your blood. They then decided I was stable and should just come back at six monthly intervals, forgetting to mention that I should be coming to the clinic for monthly blood tests, because of the medication I was taking.

During early 1997 I began feeling fatigued and tired. I had hugely swollen legs and feet from fluid retention. I was also coughing constantly – a dry tickly repetitive cough. In August we went on holiday to Cuba and had a wonderful time except I didn't have a lot of energy and just wanted to spend time reading on the beach. Walking from the beach to the hotel was an effort and I felt lazy, sluggish and generally not very enthusiastic to see this beautiful country.

At home in September 1997 I became weaker, more fatigued, legs and feet extremely swollen. I could barely walk to the end of my street; getting in and out of the car was a challenge and I couldn't cope with work. My skin had developed a yellowish tone and my eyelids were swollen – in fact I looked distinctly strange. My GP just kept giving me sick notes and telling me to rest, insisting that anaemia wasn't causing this. Many GPs never see a case of PM or DM and are totally flummoxed by it and tend to keep fobbing you off in the hope this mysterious illness is all in your imagination.

By the beginning of October I realised that within a few days I would be unable to walk and went to my GP and insisted I should see a specialist. They telephoned a hospital and I saw a rheumatologist the next day (sometimes the NHS is wonderful!).

I explained my symptoms to a charming doctor, who arranged for urine samples and blood tests and after receiving the results the next day, telephoned and arranged for me to go into hospital within 48 hours. My kidneys were leaking protein and the lining of my lungs had been scarred. My CK was 5000.

Going into hospital was quite a shock! My companions in the rheumatology ward were three ladies in their 90s – two who had dementia and one who needed assistance with her breathing. The nights were quite noisy and the days were depressing.

I was immediately prescribed 60mg prednisolone a day. This, fortunately for me, had a miraculous effect and within 3 or 4 days I felt a new woman. The water retention disappeared – what a way to lose weight; I was a stone lighter within a week (to come back later after a few weeks of steroid therapy!) My cough disappeared. I had all the tests within those two weeks, including the wonderfully unforgettable experience of a muscle biopsy (all of you who have experienced this will know what I mean).

Back at home I gradually lowered my dose of steroids over the next 18 months and had a weekly dose of 25mg of methotrexate. All seemed well for a while, until in September 1999 my CK started rising from the 200 that it had been for several months. At that time I had managed to get down to around 8mg a day of prednisolone and I think that this was the problem, in that this was too low a dose. By March 2000 my CK was 2000. My rheumatologist had by then increased my prednisolone to 20mg. There was no change in my condition for the next year and I was feeling weak, tired and bloated with steroids.

In June 2001 I decided, for health reasons to avoid having cows' milk, because I believed, having read an excellent book by Professor Jane Plant, that it could be associated with breast and prostrate cancer. I have now replaced butter and milk with soya. Initially, tea did taste a little odd but I got used to it and managed to persuade my husband to do the same; he had the added bonus of losing a few pounds because he wasn't eating so much yoghurt.

In October 2001, my CK decreased to 1250 and I began to feel much stronger and was coughing less. I have no idea whether dropping dairy produce from my diet had anything to do with my improved condition. I do think that diet can play an important part in this illness though and that dropping dairy produce and wheat from your diet may well be worth trying. My doctor reduced the steroids to 12.5 mg as well as continuing with the methotrexate. Since then my CK decreased to around 400 and I could actually run up the stairs. I remained stable for about a year and then began coughing almost constantly. My CK doubled to 800. I went to see a lung specialist who is now looking at ways to stop the interstitial lung disease, which has in fact worsened over the last 18 months. PM may also affect organs, such as heart, lungs and kidneys as well as muscles.

So, the story about my illness has not ended. Perhaps the biggest downside of this illness is all the highs and lows. Just as you are beginning to feel well and are recovering and you have a period of stability, it can flare up again. Also, most of us look very healthy and it is not really obvious that we have an illness. The condition is so rare that no one has heard of it, which means that friends constantly forget you have an illness. When you need a little sympathy and understanding it's hard to be told that everybody gets tired these days because of the pace of life!

I have, however, managed to lead a fairly normal life over the last few years, whereas I know that many fellow sufferers have had to give up their jobs and are now housebound, so for that, I am grateful. I am also very lucky to have two excellent doctors who are looking after me, even though they haven't got a clue what is the cause of this disease and are uncertain as to how I will react to their various remedies.

I have tried in the past, acupuncture and homeopathy, and perhaps should have carried on with these remedies longer to give them a chance. I know people who are being treated with alternative remedies such as Chinese herbalism, acupuncture, etc. but feel that, for me it would be too risky to go along that road at the moment, particularly as my lungs are involved.

I am, however, optimistic about the future and as more and more specialists are having to deal with sufferers they will hopefully pool their knowledge and research and find remedies other than steroids.

Update

It's now April 2005 and I have been stable for the last 18 months. This has been effected by the introduction of cyclosporin, combined with a weekly dose of methotrexate. As a consequence I have been able to slowly reduce the prednisolone and am now steroid free. My CK level has been around 90-120 for the last 6 months.

Side effects are regular stomach upsets because as a result of the medication I cannot tolerate acidic foods and I do suffer more with pains in my joints and of course have less energy. However, it's all worth it, not to have to take steroids. I am still working full-time and am in my mid fifties so that's another reason I probably have less energy.

I can now walk around 3-4 miles without getting too exhausted and this is a huge improvement. There has been no change in my lung condition for the last two years.

I do worry what the long term side effects will be from taking this combination of NSAIDS. However, for now, I am very happy to be leading a normal life.

Adrienne   PM
44 years old. Diagnosed aged 38

Rules – The one rule is that there are no rules in this disease; we are all different although we bear many similarities.

I was diagnosed officially in 2000 with polymyositis/overlapped with scleroderma & Raynauds. I was 38 and had a pressured job and young son. Slowly I felt I was losing grip on everything.

It started with itchy skin which they diagnosed as eczema. I knew different. I knew something bad was happening. We know deep down when something is not right. My consultant tried to give me azathioprine. I was not happy with this. After reading the leaflet, I was more concerned about the tablets than the disease that was creeping up on me. Steroids were a no. I had taken these two years before for 3 weeks and did not get on well with them at all. I think one of the things that made me question what was going on around me with medication was the lack of explanation one gets. Because of the overlap could this tablet help both diseases?

Gradually, over the first year I went from a strong woman, never stopping, playing with my son and most importantly shopping, to the agility of an old woman. I had trained in the gym/aerobics more than three times a week and now I could not even play football with my son. Not only was the weakness problematic, but because of the fact that the skin on my body was tightening, I was not able to stretch. One thought that always sticks in my mind is when I tried to turn over in bed at night, I felt I was wearing a baby romper suit that was too small.

It was like having Chinese burns when you tried to stretch the skin. My hands were going purple in shops so I started to wear gloves for the warmth and the grip. I couldn't hold doors open and trying to get up stairs was a task. Trying to get people around me to understand what was happening was the most difficult thing. My skin had only slightly changed and therefore I looked fairly normal. People have to live with you to be aware of how you do things and the things you can't do.

I did not understand my tests at first but I got the hang of it all after the net research I did. They say it is bad to research on the net but I feel it helps to know what is going on. It is your life and you are responsible for it. My CK was going up and up (990) and I had a problem with my heart muscle which had been affected by the myositis. I could not walk far and was out of breath. I could not run or do anything I used to be able to do. I couldn't cook potatoes without someone holding the pot, all my independence had been whisked from under my feet.

I decided to try and combat this disease without drugs. It is a choice we all are able to make and I am not saying it is the right one, just the one I wanted to take. I had to go to a new consultant and they would not see me if I did not go on any form of treatment; this was a tricky one. I wanted to try for a baby so they suggested IVIG as this was safe if you wanted to get pregnant. I had two lots and was supposed to have them every three months but this did not happen for some reason. On my second one I was very ill afterwards; in fact worse than when I went in. This cleared in about a week or two and then I felt a little better. I believe this treatment mops up the disease, but only temporarily.

I tried many other alternative routes to no avail. The acupuncture was too painful because the skin and muscles were so tender, although I did keep it up for a short time. I decided to go with the pace of life I had been given so I accepted the slowness and the loss of strength etc.

I am 5 or 6 years down the line now and my CK is going down slowly (180). I have good and bad days. I think in my case the mental aspect of this disease is so important. If you are happy then you seem to feel better. I was suffering from depression. I am not sure whether it came before, with or after the disease and once again was being offered anti-depressants. Once again I opted not to go down that road. I was sent to a psychologist who I am working with at present dealing with the anger against this monster that has taken over my life. I have come to accept my speed and capabilities in life now and go with them. If I feel good then I do more, if I don't I rest. I have suffered all the different effects that you get with this disease, the tenderness, weight loss, loss of strength, itchy skin, red blotches, pains in the chest, breathing problems, swallowing problems, tight skin. None of them has made me want to go through the side effects of the drugs. Maybe as you recall I knew in the beginning I had something seriously wrong so in the same way I knew I did not have to take the drugs? No I do not have a high tolerance level for pain. When something is new and you don't know what to expect it is easier to accept and endure it. As you get to know the pain it becomes less acceptable so I will never say never and neither should you!

Vanessa   PM
36 years old. Diagnosed aged 28

I was diagnosed with polymyositis back in December of 1997. At the time the rheumatologists thought it was a mixed connective tissue disease combining polymyositis with probably scleroderma but since then they have settled on myositis.

Looking back I had symptoms from around the summer of 1995 when I started to feel fatigued following various infections (including bronchitis and gastroenteritis) that had been treated with repeated courses of antibiotics. In the autumn of 1995 I moved up to Newcastle upon Tyne and started a full time job as a lecturer at the university. I think that the stress of moving, coping with a demanding work environment with long hours and another bout of gastroenteritis precipitated the development of the myositis. I started to feel increasingly tired from the December of 1996 until it got to the point where climbing the stairs to my upstairs Tyneside flat was a challenge. I had a multitude of aches and pains in my muscles and joints, chest pain when it was cold, developed difficulties swallowing and started to experience violent episodes of diarrhoea and vomiting after large meals. Going to restaurants was no longer a pleasure. Being half French this was most disconcerting!

For a year I had been seen by a hand specialist as I was finding it difficult to grip and close my fingers. I saw various baffled physiotherapists and a surgeon who was convinced I had Dupuytren's contraction. As this is more common among middle aged alcoholic men I was unconvinced and saw a rheumatologist in France who urged me not to have surgery but to see a rheumatologist back in Britain. I found myself on a long waiting list and waited. In the meantime my GP got me in to see a gastroenterologist who asked the right questions and tested my CK. Suddenly a rheumatologist materialised asking why I hadn't been to see them (!) and I've been under their care ever since at a hospital in Newcastle.

The main treatment I've received is oral prednisolone with doses varying from 10mg to 60mg daily. Whenever we've tried to go below 10mg I've had a relapse. My CK during a flare rises to around 2,000 and is deemed normal at around 150. A couple of years ago I tried azathioprine as a steroid sparing agent but the side effects proved too much. From low level nausea they developed to constant clusters of mouth ulcers and vomiting up to five times a day. I lost a lot of weight and felt very drained. I ended up taking my first protracted period of sick leave from work, ironically not because of the polymyositis itself but the effects of the medication. In contrast to the reaction I had to azathioprine I have been very lucky so far with the prednisolone. Apart from having to take care of my bones due to increased risk of osteoporosis, which runs in my family anyway, I've avoided most of the dreaded side effects. On high doses I do get the rounded cheeks which led one close friend to dub me the anorexic hamster as I've got thinner in general! I also get the dry skin but baby oil, shea and cocoa butter take care of that.

Over the years various other medications have been added to the mix. I've taken a variety of antacids before settling on the proton pump inhibitor lansoprazole. I'd never had acid indigestion before polymyositis so swallowing Gaviscon by the bottle was a new experience… I have learned to sleep supported by a wedge and to stay upright after meals. My gut has become the most difficult aspect of this to manage as my intestines and bowels have slowed right down to occasionally comatose levels. The resulting constipation, abdominal distension to the point of looking heavily pregnant, then overflow diarrhoea and faecal incontinence is proving a puzzler for my gastro consultant who, after many tests for other conditions such as pancreatitis and bacterial overgrowth, has settled for the line: "it's the polymyositis". Motility drugs have proved useless or had the unfortunate side effect of turning me into a zombie. I have found that avoiding overly fatty foods and dairy helps, as does trying to remain as stress free as possible. However, this remains the most unpredictable part of my polymyositis experience. It's also an aspect which seems to be rarely discussed perhaps due to the embarrassment factor but the pattern of weakness in muscles would seem to make sense.

Recently I had the biggest flare I've ever had with CK levels around 10,000. It started soon after I began taking a bisphosphonate for osteoporosis which I have now stopped after subsequently discussing it with other polymyositis patients from the UK and US who had serious dysphagia too after taking it. I was extremely fatigued and lost a lot of weight, crashing under six stone for the first time ever. This time I ended up in hospital receiving intravenous methylprednisolone and being fed through a naso-gastric tube. With determination and a positive attitude I came home with the NG-tube after two weeks, and ten days later it was removed. With a higher dose of prednisolone and methotrexate now added to the mix, my CK levels came back down to normal in just under two months and I can now swallow again fine. I have some swallowing exercises which I do as recommended by a speech therapist and the newsletter of the Myositis Association. With help from my personal trainer I am rebuilding strength in my muscles again and putting weight back on. However, maintaining weight has been a problem for me since I was first diagnosed. I have always been slim but the polymyositis has definitely made me thinner. Again this is an aspect that I've found difficult to get advice on, as most people seem to gain weight due to the treatment with steroids and diets are usually geared to weight loss rather than healthy weight gain. At the moment I'm under the care of a dietician and drinking plenty of protein shakes. I also started taking strontium ranelate to try to stave off the development of osteoporosis and try to keep up my intake of calcium rich food and drink.

A complication of the recent flare was that an echocardiogram showed up severely impaired left ventricular function. In other words my heart is not pumping any where near as efficiently as it should. This was a surprise to everyone, as despite having had ups and downs with the polymyositis over the years, I have always presented as relatively fit with no obvious heart symptoms. I'm now on an ace inhibitor and beta-blocker to improve the pumping function of the heart but these have the unfortunate side effect of lowering my already low blood pressure which can make me feel tired. We will have to see what the long term management of this aspect of the condition will entail and whether things improve as I come out of the flare. Fortunately for now my lungs seem to be in good health.

Apart from prescribed medication, I've tried various other treatments over the years. I've found that ginger and gingko maintain good circulation along with massage with aromatherapy oils and dry body brushing. Tincture of myrrh and herbal gargles have helped stave off throat infections and mouth ulcers (I now also take folic acid supplements). I've tried various supplements for digestive health but the jury is still out. That's one area where nothing so far seems to have made any dramatic change. I try to keep my skin and hair care as natural as possible to minimise the effect of harsh chemicals on dry skin and thinning hair. Keeping my hair short has helped too. It's less stressful on the scalp and less effort to style! Paraffin wax baths ease stiff hands and hot stone massages ease the whole body. I think that maintaining fitness and mobility has been important too. Even in hospital I managed to stretch my muscles out with the help of a physiotherapist. I've been working with a personal trainer who reads all the literature I find on exercise and myositis. We make sure I have well developed core strength so that I can cope better when I do have a flare.

Equally important is making time to relax and enjoy the world around. I try to reduce stress although I'm coming to realise that full time work may be beyond me. The support of my colleagues, friends, long-suffering husband and cats has been invaluable. It's amazing how comforting a small furry creature snuggling up to you can be when you haven't the energy to move. Meditation, deep breathing exercise, visualisation and affirmations are all good ways to relax which can be done in bed although I also find that music, laughter and sunshine do the trick too. Lastly but not least, I'd like to mention my fellow myositis patients in the North East. Three of us get together regularly to chat, compare stories and offer support. Thanks guys!

Julie   PM
31 years old. Diagnosed aged 21

I was diagnosed with polymyositis in June 1996. Throughout the following years I have had various degrees in health. In 1998 my consultant prescribed methotrexate to try to reduce the inflammation. I still had flare ups. People on methotrexate will know that you cannot conceive a child as most probably it will be born with disabilities. I was desperate to start a family but held off for a while in the hope that my disease would go into remission, which it never did.

In 2003, my consultant began to increase my dosage of methotrexate to try to put me into remission but I began to hallucinate and this consequently gave me panic attacks. I had these for over a year and came off the methotrexate altogether as I could not cope with the side-effects. In October 2003, I became pregnant with my first child, which I lost to a miscarriage in January 2004.

We tried again and I became pregnant again in the February of that year. My consultant thought that it was very risky for my health and I was kept under close observation by the hospital.

I prayed every night that I would not lose this child as I was so desperate for a baby to love and care for.

Things went really well throughout the pregnancy. At first I was advised to rest a lot and take things easy.

As I got bigger I found that I gained more energy and my CK fell to around 1300. I was blooming.

In November 2004, I gave birth to a healthy baby girl, named Elizabeth Jayne. I had a normal delivery. Everybody was amazed at how well I had done.

Each time we look at her we thank God that she arrived to us safe and well.

I hope this story inspires others to continue their fight with the dreaded myositis.

At the moment, March 2005, I continue to suffer with this terrible disease but with a smile on my face and a beautiful baby by my side and loving partner.

Case Studies – Inclusion Body Myositis

Jean   **IBM**
68 years old

I was diagnosed with polymyositis in October 1994 at the age of 61. There had been a very gradual onset of the disease over a number of years, with increasing difficulty in rising from chairs and occasional falls. The falls had not been frequent enough to attach much significance to them (I usually attributed them to broken paving stones or badly fitting shoes!) but the main problem was an increasing difficulty in getting up again after a fall.

I generally had very good health and felt well, so it was only when I reached the stage of being unable to get up from a chair without using both arms, that I decided to seek medical help. This coincided with a move to a new area and a new GP so I made an early appointment to see him. He referred me to a specialist and after various tests, including a muscle biopsy, I was given the diagnosis of PM. I was offered treatment with immuno-suppressive drugs, but warned that there was no guarantee of a cure or even any improvement. The choice was mine – to take the treatment offered with a risk of side effects or let the disease take its course. After some thought I decided to go for the treatment. I started taking prednisolone and azathioprine, and apart from swollen ankles in hot weather and losing some of the wrinkles in my face, I had no side effects! The Creatine Kinase level dropped to within normal limits and within 12 months I was on a much lower dose of steroids. I also felt some exercise would be helpful and following the suggestion of my GP, my husband and I joined a local gym which we still go to two or three times a week.

When I was first given the diagnosis I had very mixed feelings. To be told you have a progressive condition for which there is probably no cure is quite devastating, but this news was somewhat ameliorated by the fact that there was a reason for my symptoms and the possibility at least of the deterioration being stopped. In the early days there was some improvement as the steroids had the effect of loosening up stiff joints and the exercise at the gym also improved mobility and strength and had the effect of making me feel good. It was a tremendous morale boost to be able to improve my performance and also to see that I was as good as, and better than, some who were younger than me!

Two or three years on it was obvious that the condition was getting worse as the falls in particular became more frequent, often happening for no apparent reason at all. The consultant then did another muscle biopsy and decided that the diagnosis was in fact, Inclusion Body Myositis (IBM) That was a great disappointment, as it seems this condition never responds to treatment. However, as I have apparently had no serious side effects from treatment, my consultant felt that I should continue with the drugs as they just might be slowing things down. I think reality began to sink in at this point, but it was still difficult to take in – after all, these sort of things always happen to someone else, don't they?

Nearly seven years have now passed and although I still walk, albeit with extreme care and the support of a stick and sometimes a walking trolley, my activities are becoming more limited. Social life is restricted because of the lack of suitable chairs or toilet facilities and spontaneity has gone as everything has to be planned carefully. Even then things can sometimes go awry as they did with a visit to the London Eye last year. Every detail of the journey was thought out, but we were not prepared for the disruption caused by a terrorist attack, which closed Waterloo Station! In fact, the whole day seemed to be a series of obstacles to be overcome and at the end of it we had a real sense of achievement at having survived the day and arrived home safely.

I could not manage without the help of my husband who gives me tremendous support in every way, but of course my limitations affect his life too. It also affects my adult children and their families. I am unable to look after the grandchildren on my own, because I can't lift or carry them, in case I fall. Not to mention the hazards of toys on the floor or an unexpected enthusiastic leaping hug from one of them! Gardening was a favourite hobby of mine, but now that is somewhat restricted and I seem to spend more time giving orders than actually getting my hands dirty!

As a Christian I firmly believe that God has a plan for my life, but I have big questions now which are not easily answered. This does not make the situation any easier, but I have to hang on in there and trust God, because whatever the circumstances may be I know He has never let me down in the past and so I must trust Him for the future too. I experience the care of an 'extended' family in church too and I have to learn to receive from others, although in the past I have more often been on the 'giving' side. Our small village church purchased a few chairs with arms for my benefit and I am delighted to see that others too really appreciate and make use of this provision.

All in all, life is very different now and constant adjustments have to be made. Many of the things we had expected to do in our retirement are not possible, but we are still able to enjoy many things together. I don't think I will ever totally get used to the fact that I can no longer go for a brisk walk in the fresh air. But I have learnt to enjoy a drive in the car round our beautiful Oxfordshire villages and to sit in the car and look at the sea while my husband takes a walk. I have experienced much kindness from family, friends and health care professionals and I have realised how little understanding I have had in the past of the needs of people with physical disabilities. I have developed a new skill in writing letters and become something of a campaigner for the needs of the disabled. This in itself can be very rewarding when I get a positive response, but it needs determination at times to keep up the campaign. Many local events take place in schools, with small chairs, or churches and village halls which are in desperate need of modernisation. Even shops are slow to change in spite of new legislation. When I mentioned to one shopkeeper that the step at the entrance was so high that my husband had to give me a push to get up it, he replied, 'It's been like that since 1862 madam and no one has ever complained before'. At times like this you can only see the funny side of the situation and be thankful for others who are more thoughtful.

Although I do get very tired at times I do not have any pain and generally feel well, for this I am very thankful. However, this does cause frustration when I can't do the things I feel I would like to do and the fact that I usually look well makes it difficult to explain to people why I seem so strangely helpless at times. The opportunity to meet and talk with others who have the same problems is a tremendous help. It is such a relief not to be the 'odd one out' with this strange condition and to know that others are experiencing the same problems.

It is sometimes a difficult balancing act to accept and adjust to what cannot be changed and yet not give up, but keep on with the battle.

Update

When Jenny wrote and asked me to add to my story I was not sure what I could say that would be helpful and interesting. As the muscle weakness has gradually increased we have had to continue to adapt in various ways; we have installed a stair lift in our house, put in a bathroom with a level access shower and bought a comfortable wheelchair (which I can get out of!) to give us the opportunity to go for longer 'walks' and also to provide my own seating when going to places where there are no chairs with arms.

Then the unexpected happened. Whilst out shopping one day I fell (as we do from time to time!) and this time, instead of a few bruises or a sprained ankle, I suffered a fracture of the neck of the femur which was repaired with a partial hip replacement. The operation was very successful and initial recovery quite quick. However, the worst part of all this was the fact that nobody apart from the physiotherapist, seemed to have heard of myositis. It was hard work trying to explain, while suffering from shock and in pain, why I had difficulty in moving the undamaged leg – which actually happened to be my weakest one.

After the operation I was put on a pressure mattress, which may be ideal for preventing bedsores but as I had no firm base on which to push myself up, it meant I was totally helpless and needed two nurses to lift me up even to get a drink. I was quite sure I would be better off without this mattress, but I had great difficulty in persuading the nurs-

ing staff to remove it. When they eventually did they were amazed to discover that this apparently helpless woman was now able to do things for herself and decided that perhaps she did know what she was taking about! The bedside chair was not quite high enough for me to get out of unaided, so my husband brought in a 'lift-up' cushion from home. Again, no one had ever seen anything like it but they were delighted that their work load was lightened. The final problem was the need for two people to lift me from the commode in a ward which was very short staffed. I don't need to go into details about this situation. When I told the staff that I had a catalogue at home which advertised adjustable height commodes they contacted the Occupational Therapist who managed to find one for me to use. After all that they decided that the best thing was to send me home as soon as possible. Of course, I was delighted and I hope that one or two doctors and nurses are now a little more aware of some of our problems.

I am now waiting for physiotherapy and a little uncertain about the future, as the risk of falling seems to be something we have to live with. Living with myositis certainly means constant adjustment in life-style and keeping on with the battle.

Frank   IBM
79 years old

During the 5 years which it took to diagnose IBM, I met with local total ignorance of the disease, local professional incompetence and administrative chaos at my hospital. Eventually at a Southampton hospital I found an efficient, knowledgeable and helpful service.

October 1995
Total right knee replacement due to osteoarthritis.

January 1996
Began to fall.

January 1996/December 1998
Physiotherapy. Given exercises to do. Despite my assertions that my condition was deteriorating I was twice discharged as cured.

July 1999
Saw a locum doctor. Referred to hospital.

January 2000
Saw an Orthopaedic consultant. Referred to a neurophysical consultant.

July 2000
Saw neurophysical consultant. Nothing wrong. Said I should see a neurological consultant.

July 2000
Discharged.

July 2000
The locum doctor referred me back to a neurological consultant.

August 2000
Saw neurological consultant. Referred me to a Neurological Unit.

October 2000
Saw neurologist – suspected IBM

December 2000
Biopsy – due to 80% wastage on my thigh muscle, specimen was taken from my arm.

January 2001
IBM confirmed!

During this period I met with an enormous amount of frustration, which resulted in a great deal of telephoning and writing. I have quite a bulky file!

Update

After I was diagnosed with IBM in 2001, I was transferred back to the care of my GP. As there was no known cure he and his ancillary staff offered no help, advice or treatment and because my health is good for an 82 year old, I have not seen my GP for some 18 months. My information and news has come from the Myositis Support Group and the Internet.

Initially I got about with a walking stick and my wife's arm but stairs were a problem. In January 2002 I lost my concentration and my footing and fell backwards down the stairs, knocking myself out. I was rushed to A & E where, after a cursory examination, a doctor said nothing was wrong and I was sent home. Two weeks later I blacked out and I was taken back to A & E where a scan revealed a sub dural haematoma (blood clot on the brain). After two weeks I was removed to another hospital. By noon the next day I was down in the operation suite. I came to in a ward with three drainage tubes in my head. After ten days I was sent home.

From then on I have taken extreme care and this may be a contributory factor in my increasing disability. I now use two crutches and a wheeled walker. Getting up from chairs, meals out and theatre visits are no go areas, as is public transport. I still drive my car, subject to health checks, but only locally and with extreme care. Social Services have been helpful within their cash limitations, providing small items, hand rails and grabs. I have bought stair lifts, a wheelchair (not yet used), a walker and a bath non electric riser seat and a portable chair riser seat, both of which I regard as best buys.

I find that frustration and depression are my worst enemies. It is hard watching my wife (carer) struggle with jobs which I used to do. Sometimes I wonder if all the struggling is worth while. Then I look out of my window on a sunny Spring morning and see the fields turning green, the cattle feeding, the birds busy nest building, the flowers in bloom and the blossom on the trees and I decide that it is.

Female   **IBM/Overlap**
50 years old

Having myositis has made me think a lot about the relationship between the mind and body.

I am 50 years old and have been suffering from lupus/IBM (first diagnosed as PM) for over twenty years.

When I was 17 and going out to work for the first time I was struck by the fact that compared to the families of people I met at work, my family were fortunate to enjoy good health. I felt that the situation could not last and that inevitably one of us would become ill. The thought came to me that one day I may be unable to walk.

I felt that however awful the thought of being in a wheelchair was, I would be able to cope with it. I decided that from that time onwards I would always appreciate the fact that I could walk, run and dance because some day I might not be able to. I reckoned that it would be easier for me to cope with being disabled if I learnt not to take my legs for granted.

At 17 I was in good health. By my late 20's I had been diagnosed with lupus but was not seriously affected. However, over time I began to notice that my legs had become weaker and that I was not able to do things that less fit and more overweight friends could do. I had difficulty cycling up slight slopes. I enjoyed sailing but ended up flat on my face every time I jumped off the boat. I found myself marvelling at people who could climb onto a platform or stage simply by placing one foot on it.

I had been attending a lupus clinic for many years but the doctors (after pushing on my legs a few times) kept telling me that there was no sign of weakness. Eventually I decided to write to the doctor describing what I looked like heaving my body up a flight of stairs. The message finally got through and I had a series of tests which confirmed that I had polymyositis. It was not explained to me that this was a separate condition from lupus and no treatment was offered.

I attended the clinic twice a year and my party piece was to squat in front of the doctor to show the medical students that I could not get up. Eventually I was unable to squat at all and I was worried that my useful life as a patient was coming to an end.

I was advised by a doctor friend to transfer to a different hospital where thorough investigations were carried out and the current most effective treatment was offered (prednisolone, methotrexate and azathioprine). Unfortunately there was no improvement. Subsequent further tests showed that the correct diagnosis was in fact IBM.

Each year my legs are a little weaker and my life becomes a little more restricted. I believe that Western medicine cannot offer me anything further – although I am very grateful to the doctors who have tried to help me. I now tend to pursue either Chinese medicine or homeopathy.

I have seen nutritionists in the past and tried other alternative treatment offered by both healers and charlatans. I have spent a fortune trying to distinguish between the two. However I do believe from my experience that food intolerance and the functioning of the gut do have an important role to play in myositis and I am continuing to explore this area.

I am also aware that at 17 years old I had a gut feeling that something was going to happen to me, which in fact did happen. I am sure that appreciating my legs when they functioned well has helped me to cope with the effects of my disability.

However, I have not yet reached a conclusion as to whether I predicted my illness, whether my thoughts sent messages to my body which caused the illness or whether it is all just a coincidence.

Update

In the last three years IBM has caused my life to change radically. Every year for the past twenty five years I have become slightly weaker, but I have now reached a stage where every small deterioration has a significant impact on my ability to function.

I found that my work was exhausting me but I worried about admitting it as I was scared that I would be forced to work part-time which I could not afford to do. Luckily I had a sympathetic Occupational Health doctor who recommended me for medical retirement and I received excellent advice on benefits from the local Disabled Association, so the financial impact was not too drastic.

I feel so much better now that I can control my day and although my muscles are weak – I no longer suffer from fatigue.

I have had difficulty in climbing stairs for years but last year I suddenly found that I was unable to do so at all. I accepted this as an inevitable deterioration in my illness. Soon after I found I had difficulty driving and could barely get out of my car. I then fell and broke my knee cap. I recovered well once my legs were out of plaster (which was an extremely difficult time) but by this time I had lost my confidence and became very reclusive.

I fell into the trap of thinking that because IBM is incurable, there was no possibility of any improvement. However, when I found I was too afraid to go out into my garden I contacted the physiotherapy department and begged for an appointment. I have always had an exercise routine but the physiotherapists gave me exercises to stimulate muscles that have atrophied through lack of use (as opposed to disease). Now I have regained enough strength and confidence to go out on my own. The next time I have a sudden decline I will request another physiotherapy appointment and not regard it as an inevitable decline in my condition.

Female   **IBM**
58 years old

Although my myositis was diagnosed in Autumn 1996 I believe that I have actually suffered from the condition for about thirteen years.

The onset was insidious: I was aware of feeling extremely tired but was not conscious of being ill. I thought that it was possibly part of the ageing process although I was only in my forties and had always been relatively active and fit. I joined a keep fit class which of course, was not helpful at all as I felt exhausted after each session.

Over a period of approximately five years I developed considerable weakness in my legs and pelvic girdle, arms and shoulder girdle, and hands. Wasting of my forearms also became apparent (my watch strap was becoming loose). The left side of my body was more affected than my right side. I also experienced dysphagia (difficulty with swallowing) which was particularly noticeable when I ate dense food such as bread. I also noticed that my balance was not good.

Because the disease was progressing slowly, I was beginning to accommodate the symptoms and avoided activities which were becoming more difficult. I was still unaware that I was ill but certainly felt that all was not as it should be. I was unable to rise from the squat position and gripping items with my left hand was difficult. I also had three inexplicable falls. Climbing the stairs was possible but not easy and walking uphill was even more arduous. I discovered however, that by leaning forward as I walked helped.

In 1996, I was referred to my local teaching hospital where I was fortunate to see a neurologist who recognised that I had quite a problem and immediately arranged for me to undergo the necessary investigations: an electromyogram, blood tests and a muscle biopsy. Even at this early stage the possibility of a second opinion was mentioned.

The tests revealed a raised creatine kinase, the EMG indicated muscle disease and the muscle biopsy showed areas of severe inflammation. A diagnosis of polymyositis was given and a regime of high dose steroids together with an immunosuppressant started. Unfortunately, I reacted very badly to the steroids and consequently they were withdrawn, slowly, after only a few months. I did, however, continue to take the immunosuppressants.

Meanwhile, the wasting of my left arm was increasing and my hand and fingers felt weak. My neck, shoulder girdle and pelvic girdle were also weak but I think that my swallowing at that point had improved a little.

After a period of observation, I was referred to a rheumatologist for a second opinion and inclusion body myositis was mentioned for the first time. A second muscle biopsy proved to be inconclusive although my creatine kinase continued to be raised.

A third opinion was then sought from a different neurologist at the same hospital and I underwent another electromyogram and yet a further muscle biopsy. The EMG still suggested muscle disease and the muscle biopsy remained inconclusive but despite this, a clinical diagnosis of inclusion body myositis was confirmed. Because of my dysphagia I was referred for a videofleuroscopy (a type of barium swallow) after which the speech therapist prescribed some useful exercises.

Since being diagnosed in 1996, I have received courses of various immunosuppressants some of which seem to have provided some stability of the condition and which, I feel, may even have slowed down the progression of the disease, but because of serious side effects most have had to be withdrawn. Overall my disease over the past few years has progressed, albeit slowly.

Myositis inhibits my life inasmuch as my mobility is limited and my fine motor skills impaired. This causes me great frustration but I try to find interests and activities that I am still able to pursue. Because of the inaccessibility of tube stations (there are stairs everywhere) I find that I have difficulty visiting places such as the theatre and it is necessary for me to rely on a member of the family to take me. As my knees are likely to give way at times, I fear falling so prefer to have someone with me when out shopping, and if I go out for a meal I often need help with the cutting up of food. Driving a manual car is now impossible but I shall soon acquire a car with automatic transmission and power steering and consequently regain some freedom.

It is always a difficult situation for any family when one of them becomes ill but I think that coping is made easier for everyone if the practical issues are dealt with so that independence can be maintained for as long as possible. It may even be necessary to move house. Emotionally, people deal with chronic illness in their own way and this will vary enormously. Personally, I feel that it is something to just get on with whilst at the same time remaining positive.

Inclusion body myositis is a very difficult disease to diagnose and also to treat but the progression of the disease is slow and I am grateful to receive continued treatment whilst it is still available despite the side effects.

Update

It was in spring 2003 that I first wrote about my IBM when I was still receiving treatment. In November of that year I was given a week's course of IVIG which seemed to provide more strength in my arms but not my legs.

When I next saw my consultant in January 2004, all treatment for my IBM was stopped and since that time my condition has very slowly deteriorated and as a result I have been falling over from time to time, causing a fractured toe on one occasion but generally causing tissue damage which would put me out of action for two or three weeks at a time (my knees buckle unexpectedly). I usually rely on the arm of my husband or that of a companion for support when I'm out. I find that I get tired very easily and now need help with the housework. My general weakness makes getting in and out of the bath impossible now and at night I am aware of considerable twitching in my calf muscles. Because of my weak arms, I am unable to lift my grandchildren but I still derive great pleasure from seeing them.

I miss being able to look after my garden as this was my main hobby before I became ill. I also miss being able to go for long walks in the country – something the family always did on holidays in the past.

Hopefully, at some time in the future, help will be available for people with IBM but meanwhile I do as much as I am able, accept my limitations and fortunately continue to receive the support of my family.

Jim   **IBM**
69 years old

My story begins around February 1998 when, strangely enough, aboard the liner QE2 I slipped quite dramatically down the main central staircase. At the time I thought nothing of it – it just seemed a case of carelessness. Later on, however, I came to think that this was probably the first sign that something was going wrong. Here I must add, I was in the best of health at the age of 65, already five years into retirement after 40 years of flying as a pilot with the Fleet Air Arm and subsequently two major international airlines. This entailed having no less than 80 rigorous medical checks (one every six months) to keep my licence intact – so you can see that any suggestion that anything had suddenly gone wrong was an anathema to me.

Some time afterwards I experienced a feeling of walking unsteadily, accompanied occasionally with pain and, more alarmingly, sudden and completely unexplained falls. I was still playing regular golf and tennis and also trying to manage a garden (on a hillside too!) So it was that in March 1999 I went to my GP to seek an explanation – by now the falls were becoming more frequent. I was referred to a rheumatologist, who thought my posture was to blame, recommending the filling of orthotics in the shoes to counteract my knock-kneed tendency. At the same time an x-ray confirmed two degenerate joints in the left ankle.

Also, around this time, I became aware that after 18 holes of golf I needed a half-hour nap to recover, accompanied by a distinct stiffness (almost pain) in the thighs. Again, I just put this down to age, and was not too concerned. However, the feeling of unsteady walking persisted and in November 1999 I had a spectacular double fall on holiday among coral rocks on the beach, resulting in emergency treatment at a local clinic. A friend witnessing this was amazed to see that this was no trip or stumble on an uneven surface, but a total collapse each time as if I had been pole-axed on the spot.

Returning home, I began to feel pain in the left knee and took ibuprofen regularly. My GP recommended physiotherapy, but this had no effect at all. I also had an MRI scan on the knee, which confirmed some cartilage break-up. This led to keyhole surgery to 'suck' the bits out in February 2000, which was very successful and I have had no pain there since. The surgeon also noted that I had considerable muscle loss in both thighs, this being purely a visual conclusion.

Unfortunately, this knee business turned out to be a red herring, which disguised the real cause of falling, awkward gait etc. My legs were getting progressively more tired now and golf had to be limited to nine holes, prompting a return visit to the rheumatologist. He recommended more physiotherapy, which, again, did no good (because as we now know in hindsight, muscles destroyed cannot be reinstated). He did, though, remark on the marked deterioration in the bulk or muscle mass of the quadriceps and asked to see me a few weeks later. This time he became quite concerned because a thorough check revealed even more deterioration of the quadriceps as well as a 50% loss of hand-grip on my left side. Some nerve dysfunction was suspected, and this time an MRI scan of the lower back was arranged, coupled with a nerve conduction test. The neurologist ruled out any nerve problems straight away, but the scan did show some deterioration of the lower lumbar region. Most significantly, though, the neurologist suspected a muscle problem, and even said he thought he knew what it was, but wouldn't tell me until after the result of a muscle biopsy was known. This I had in December 2000. My falling rate had reached at least one every ten days or so, the legs buckling without warning, even at home – it was impossible to say which leg was to blame, it happened so quickly.

The truth came out two weeks later in January 2001 when the biopsy revealed the presence of IBM. So at least I was spared a misleading or incorrect diagnosis as sometimes occurs with myositis. The shock took some time to sink in, but the thought that the situation was not life-threatening parried the blow somewhat. The fact that there was (and is) no cure for IBM was a hard thing to stomach. I started taking Creatine pills as a consultant said it would do no harm and might do some good. I also volunteered to take part in a Creatine trial at King's College, but had to abandon it half way through after I fractured my lower right fibula during a fall in a car park. This fracture healed very well, and I then started using a stick for the very first time. However, a painful ankle persisted for several months, and the rheumatologist said that Glucosamine might be helpful – indeed it was, and in only a short time all the pain disappeared. I still take it regularly as well as Creatine and Cod liver oil pills.

Falls still occur from time to time, often wrenching tendons and ligaments and causing much bruising. This is because one falls straight down when the buckling occurs, as if pole-axed, and the feet have no time to get out of the way before being crushed by one's own body weight. Mercifully, they are much less frequent than previously, mainly because I take more care and do things more slowly. Exercise is recommended, but I find I have to 'ration' it out. For instance, if I swim 20 lengths at the local baths in the morning, I would have to be very careful doing any gardening in the afternoon otherwise some buckling of knees would occur. Stairs are a great problem, as is getting up from cramped seating in buses, trains and planes. I avoid these if possible, though driving is no problem at present.

Needless to say, tennis had to be abandoned over two years ago and golf went the same way after I broke my leg in September 2001. Standing at functions and shows gets very tiring after an hour or so and a mile is about the maximum walking distance without rest. A portable half-step of about four inches would be useful to carry around for getting into coaches, old buildings etc, but I haven't found one yet.

I have now learned to live with IBM. My friends tell me I look well and seem remarkably cheerful about it all, but I think the reality is that I have always had a good sense of humour and this masks the deep-down feeling of 'why me?' which surfaces in quieter moments. It certainly doesn't do any good to feel morbid, and it was a great relief actually to meet people in the same boat at my first AGM of the Myositis Support Group in July 2001. As I approach my 70th birthday I have to reflect that I have been fortunate in having a good life with, hopefully, many more years to come. IBM does not seem to get the mention or the attention that other forms of myositis get, but I wish the Support Group and researchers success in their endeavours to find a cure or at least to find the cause.

Update

There has been a downward trend in my condition in the three years since I wrote my 'story'. A fall two years ago resulted in a double fracture, with six weeks in a wheelchair and three weeks wearing a 'moon-boot'. This inevitably allowed more thigh muscles to waste away. I get tired from very little exercise now and the twenty length swim has been reduced to no more than three.

A 45-minute nap in the afternoon is essential, as is a stick for walking even a few yards. Walking range is down from a mile to 300 yards or so, without fatigue. Stairs are really a big problem and I avoid any flight of more than five steps. My left-hand grip has weakened considerably and a raised toilet-seat is another 'must'.

That morbid tale of woe is, however, counterbalanced by the fact that I have far fewer falls, the average being only one every three months instead of the previous every ten days. This is due to increased care and being less adventurous. Also, I still enjoy driving without much difficulty and I still remain mainly cheerful – or so others tell me. However, I am still mystified as to why IBM cases feature so little in Buddy Lists, Bulletin Boards and Association magazines both here and in the USA. At the last UK Association meeting there was precisely one IBM sufferer apart from myself.

Joyce   **IBM**
56 years old. Diagnosed aged 49

During October, 1997 I decided, reluctantly, I really would have to visit my GP. For some time I had had niggling questions about why my walking had slowed down, why climbing steps to our front door had become more difficult, why I had experienced inexplicable falls. I tried Shiatsu massage. It was at one of these visits, I was asked when I had broken my toe. Initially I had no recollection of this happening. Later I remembered having a fall, very badly bruising my foot, nearly 5 years before. I only recall the date because it was a day out on our 20th wedding anniversary. I was shocked to realise my problems had been going on slowly all that time.

I was surprised to find the GP was a woman, I don't know why, but that sticks in my mind. I was equally surprised to find she took what I said seriously. After some strength tests, she has a slight build but was still able to resist my pushes and pulls, she suggested I needed to see a neurologist and to return for blood tests the following day.

Within 3 weeks I saw a neurologist, who said he would need to do further tests at a hospital in Plymouth. Just over a week later, on a Tuesday, I was installed in my allocated space in hospital – how did that happen? I expected it to take at least 6 months to even get on a wait-ing list for a bed! Most inconveniently my class (I'm a teacher) were mid-Christmas production rehearsals.

"Don't worry, I'll only be in 2 or 3 days, should be back in on Friday," I reassured them. I finally left hospital Friday afternoon.

"I was fine until I came in here," I joked, as I hobbled out on my crutches. I'd had a basic MOT, nerve conduction test and muscle biop-sy. I also spoke with a doctor who came up with two obscure options, that I either had polymyositis or inclusion body myositis. He suspect-ed the latter and warned me that there was no treatment. Needless to say at the time neither option meant anything to me.

It was not until the end of January, a few weeks after my 49th birth-day, the diagnosis of IBM was confirmed. I took the attitude of it just being a label. I was no different walking out of that consulting room with the name of this disease written on a piece of paper (I'd never remember what it was called) than I was when I'd walked in.

About a week or two later, I visited my GP, having come up with dozens of questions, what was I supposed to do now? She has been so incredibly supportive. Her honesty about having little knowledge of IBM was daunting but she had a willingness to share in finding out. She then moved to another local practice and it was a great relief that I managed to do the same some time later. I need to see her infre-quently but totally trust in her support.

Initially I had an excellent physiotherapist who visited me at home. She left the post a few years ago, re-organisation meant her position was not filled and the system has now changed. I also had some sup-port from an occupational therapist but I have been unable to contact her recently, so don't know what the position is there.

I took early retirement from teaching. I just couldn't keep up. Some things I couldn't do at all, e.g. move P.E. equipment, rearrange classroom furniture, carry around piles of books, take my turn on playground duty, help young children with coats and laces…etc…etc., all important parts of being in a primary school. To this day, I miss being there……….

Moving house was the next major hurdle. Finding a property with level access in hilly Paignton was no easy task. We did find this bunga-low though and spent a lot of money changing the bathroom to a wetroom, re-building the front to provide a ramp and take away a step inside, re-build a lean-to bit in the kitchen to level the floor and re-fit the kitchen.

I then devoted a lot of time doing voluntary work with a national charity helpline for children. I thoroughly enjoyed it and even did a parachute jump to raise funds. I couldn't get up a flight of steps but was able to jump out of an aeroplane! I worked with an amazing, committed, great bunch of people. I also did drug trials at Kings College with an excellent doctor who really actually knew about IBM, a rare find indeed!

My specialist now works mainly with MS patients so I have a new one. My new neurologist, I'm sure, is excellent but there is so little to offer I wonder why I take up his time. I can no longer get access to my place of voluntary work and other problems have arisen there which have been very difficult to deal with. My husband and I separated and my son is very happy enjoying a new life with his partner. My future prospects seem more uncertain than ever.

I think it is really important to recognise that apart from the physical difficulties, the mental and emotional traumas can sometimes be overwhelming. It's great to read and hear the fantastic things people do and the way they cope but, for me there needs to be a balance, so I know I'm not the only one who struggles sometimes, that everyone has their ups and downs.

Of all the stories I have read about people with IBM, I have never heard of such a direct clear cut arrival at the diagnoses as my own. To this day I am still amazed at my first specialist making his diagnosis so quickly. I am still able to get around with the aid of a stick and my AFOs – ankle and foot ortheses – never leave home without them! The very slow progress with improving access to places is frustrating but at least something is beginning. I can understand how difficult it is for many people to have any concept of the problems even a few steps can have.

At the last Myositis Association Conference in Birmingham, I met a few other people with IBM, so it was brilliant. I look forward to being at the next one, if I can still travel to it! The isolation of being an IBM sufferer is difficult, so to hear other people speaking about it is something of a relief. I would like to hope everyone reading this book will find lots of love, happiness and peace of mind.

Valerie   **IBM**
39 years old. Diagnosed aged 33

I was diagnosed with IBM in October 1999 after many years of not knowing what was going wrong with my body. It all started back in 1997. I was
diagnosed with ITP (a blood disorder to do with white blood cells attacking the red blood cells) and also my platelet count was very low. I was put
in hospital for nearly two weeks and started on a large dose of steroids
which continued for months. When I started to come off the steroids I
started to feel that my legs were feeling a little weak, but I didn't think too
much about it at the time. I was working at a residential home for the
elderly and it involved a lot of walking and running up and down stairs.

After a little while I noticed more weakness and then I started to fall
for no apparent reason. I went to see my GP and was just told to keep
my weight down and my legs would be alright. I left it for another few
months but I found I was falling more frequently and also that I could-
n't get up very easily. I went to see another GP.

He referred me to the neurology department at our local hospital
but it took six months before my appointment came through. Then in
October 1999 I spent two weeks in hospital and had lots of different
tests. The muscle biopsy found that I had Inclusion Body Myositis.

At the time, I was three months pregnant with my youngest child
and my doctor didn't want to start me on any medication. However, he
decided to go ahead with steroids. When my daughter was two months
old my doctor started me on a course of methotrexate. Today I am still
on methotrexate but I stopped the steroids a couple of years ago.

My arms are also becoming very weak and trying to keep up with
three active children from five to fourteen years old is not easy. Since
the day I was told about the disease and the way that things will go in
time, I feel very scared. Every day I try to keep on my feet, but it is hard
not to think of the future with three children who are still quite young.

Graham   **IBM**
55 years old. Diagnosed aged 45

The first time I remember something was not quite right was in 1995
when I was 45. I was on holiday in Cornwall with my family. One
evening, whilst they went off to do something else, I decided to go sea

fishing in this beautiful cove I'd found. This necessitated a climb down a small cliff, no problem so far. I was there for a couple of hours until the tide came in, time to go. I started to climb back up the cliff. My god, did I struggle. My legs didn't seem to have the power I normally had to lift myself up. I finally made it to the top and put the episode down to needing to loose some weight, and perhaps my age.

As time went on I noticed increasingly similar problems going up stairs at home and the office (in my youth I would vault up the stairs often two at a time). I also noticed my energy levels deteriorating, as well as the occasional unexplained trip that I could not recover from, ending up with me on the ground.

Putting this all down to being overweight, I lost $1\frac{1}{2}$ stone. This didn't make any difference.

At this stage I should point out that the job I had was very demanding. I was Head of Marketing for the company I worked for, plus I was on the management team running the business. Often long hours, lots of pressure, constantly working against deadlines.

The next event happened at an exhibition in London. I had organised a stand for the company and was manning it with my team. As the day wore on I progressively started to feel really ill, so much so that I ended up in the sick bay. I could not even stand because I was so disorientated, dizzy and weak. Finally, I was taken home.

The first diagnosis was that I had had a heart attack (frightening for my wife, but I was out of it at the time so did not know what was going on). Then the doctor diagnosed labyrinthitis, which is an infection of the inner ear caused by a virus.

Could this have been the problem all along?

It took more than a year to get over the worst of the labyrinthitis, but the physical tiredness and weakness remained and continued to get worse, plus the falls started to be more frequent.

In mid 1997 I decided to see my GP who passed me on through a trail of 'specialists', including one who accused me of malingering to get off work – I could have thumped him.

Finally I got diagnosed with polymyositis, but they were still unsure. This was mid 1998 and at this time my CPK level was around 1400.

I was then put under a rheumatologist and so started several years of tests, different drugs and treatments including IVIG, two biopsies and countless EMGs.

While all this treatment was going on, in an effort to find out more about polymyositis, I joined the Myositis Support Group. This was of great help to know I was not alone, as well as to get useful information about the disease.

I also started taking more control of the situation and started pursuing alternative medicines.

I visited a homeopath recommended to me, who put me on drops and suggested I started taking Co-Enzyme Q10s. This definitely improved my energy levels, particularly the Co-E Q10s and although my strength did not improve, I certainly did not feel as physically tired. I also felt better in myself.

While all this was going on my CPK lowered, varying between 700 to 900.

The homeopath also diagnosed I had a wheat intolerance, but we did not know how it was manifesting, as there were none of the normal symptoms associated with wheat intolerance.

In September 2000 one of my bloodtests showed I was developing neutropenia. This is a deficiency in the white blood cells, which reduces the ability for the body to fight off infections. Wounds to the skin also take a long time to heal.

This was all I needed.

I saw a haematologist, a really nice chap, very thorough and friendly. He was unsure whether there was a connection with my myositis. Personally I do not believe in those sorts of coincidences. Various tests ensued including my bone marrow which appeared to be OK. It was decided I would be put under observation to see how things developed. No drugs were prescribed.

By now the falls were getting worse; two to three a week were not uncommon. Typically I would be walking along and suddenly the strength in my legs would disappear – it was if someone had flicked my strength switch off. Often I would crumple to the ground and in the most awkward of ways. This would damage my legs, my ankles and tear ligaments. I would hit my head on the ground – I was doing loads of damage to myself. There was also the reaction from people seeing me fall. Comments were made that I must have been drunk, which was ironic because I hardly drink alcohol.

In March 2001, my doctor suggested I took 6 weeks off work to see if somehow the pressure of work was associated with the falls. My wife and I decided to go away for a week. Very relaxing, but still the falls continued.

Then it dawned on me, could the intolerance to wheat be causing the falls (I subsequently found out that the meridian line from the stomach goes through the leg muscles).

I immediately went onto a strict wheat avoidance diet and amazingly the type of falls where my strength suddenly switch off, stopped.

To this day I still do get the occasional fall, but generally this is because I have stepped on or down something that I was not prepared for. My falls now are something like two to three a year, not a week.

By joining the Myositis Support Group and within that, the London Support Group, I had gathered a lot of information. In mid 2001, I became increasingly suspicious that I was showing all the symptoms of inclusion body myositis not polymyositis.

This theory came to a head in October 2001. By now I had gone the full round of drug treatments including a second dose of immunoglobulin transfusion, but still remained on a base dose of steroids. Nothing was working, although my CPK was steady at around 600-700.

I passed on my suspicions to my rheumatologist who organised a third but deeper biopsy and also another EMG. However he was still unsure, but as there was nothing more he could offer me, he referred me to an IBM specialist at Kings College, London.

On the alternative medicine front I had added regular sessions of acupuncture to the homeopathic drops treatment. Whilst this was not providing a cure, generally in myself I felt reasonably OK. I could still cope with a long working day and I could still just about manage stairs etc.

Tracking back my medical history, my acupuncturist also suspected that the original virus infection had started when I had a second bout of mumps in the early 90s, which then surfaced again with the labyrinthitis, finally manifesting into myositis. She suspected the virus was still deep in my body.

I saw the specialist at Kings in November 2001. He immediately confirmed I had IBM. As none of the drugs had worked he suggested I now came off the steroids completely, which I was keen to do anyway.

He also wanted me 'clean' in preparation for some expected trials later in the year.

Unfortunately, as I gradually came off the steroids, I felt myself rapidly deteriorating. This was confirmed by my CPK climbing to nearly 2000. I was told this might happen, so I toughed it out, keen not to go back on the steroids.

My rapid deterioration also made me reconsider my situation at work. I approached my Managing Director as to whether I could step down as Head of Department, but still keep working and take on a less demanding role. This he agreed to.

In February 2002, my acupuncturist, observing my deterioration as well as a lot of heat in my body, suggested I tried traditional Chinese herbal medicine. She took me to see a doctor in London's China Town, a respected Chinese doctor well known for her work with children at Great Ormond Street Hospital.

After listening to my problem and viewing my symptoms, she checked my body rhythm and looked at my tongue. I then went for a blood test. When I returned she checked the results and prescribed about 10 herbs to be taken in the form of a tea which I would brew up each night.

The first few cups were pretty unpalatable, but after a short time I got used to them.

Every six to eight weeks the doctor required I had a blood test to check liver function and also see how things were progressing. She would adjust the ingredients based on how my body reacted.

Over the next 18 months, my CPK started to slowly reduce settling at around 1000. My neutropenia also started showing some signs of improvement, and all this was without any drugs.

Although my strength did not improve, my deterioration greatly slowed to being just moderately detectable.

I still continued with the homeopathy and acupuncture, which some might view as OTT, but I was determined to try anything. On the odd occasion I had stopped taking the homeopathic drops for more than 5 days because I had run out, I would notice deterioration. And I knew the Chinese herbs were doing me good.

To make things easier in October 2002 we moved into a bungalow.

Unfortunately on the eve of the move, I had a nasty fall whilst over-reaching and fell on my knees onto a concrete floor. I ended up in casualty for the night with a fractured kneecap.

At work, stairs were becoming do-able but difficult. Things came to a head in December 2002 when almost at the top, my leg (the one I had fractured the kneecap) had had enough and I fell, sliding down-stairs headfirst on my back. Needless to say I got banned from using the stairs.

In spring 2003 I started to work from home.

At the end of 2003, my acupuncturist gave up work to have a sec-ond child. As there was no satisfactory replacement, the acupuncture stopped. I continued with the homeopathy and Chinese herbal medi-cine, which I'm still on whilst I write this piece (March 2005).

Nothing has really changed much since except that my neutropenia is back to normal, which is marvellous. My CPK has risen slightly in the past twelve months to around 1300, which I suspect is due to dropping the acupuncture. I plan to resume this shortly.

Fortunately I'm still working, albeit from home and only 4 days a week. I certainly would not be able to afford the alternative medicines if I was not working, and I suspect, that if it was not for the alternative medicine I would not be able to work – so a 'Catch 22' situation.

Myositis is a very frightening and frustrating disease, especially if you have IBM for which there is no cure as yet. However, joining the Myositis Support Group and meeting people in a similar situation has helped me cope and find out more information about IBM. As a con-sequence, I'm not as frightened of the disease. Fortunately, I'm also not a person who gives up easily and a positive attitude has helped me through the tough times.

Has the alternative medicines helped? I can only answer for myself. I firmly believe that if I had not gone down this route, I would be in a far worst state than I am now. I can cope with a full day's work. I can be on my feet for up to 6 hours (providing the ground is flat and sta-ble). I can drive to my daughter's home and back in a day (360 miles round trip) and not bat an eyelid. Plus the alternative medicine has given me a reason to fight.

OK, I'm still deteriorating, be it extremely slowly. My strength is way down and my muscles have visibly wasted. I just don't 'do' stairs and steps, and I avoid steep slopes (why are some of these wheelchair ramps so steep?), but I keep going and am enjoying life the best I can. I've learnt to adapt, to make the most of what I can do, rather than dwell on what I can't. I've bought or made aids to help me (there's a lot out there, thank heavens for the Internet), and when things have become more difficult, I've found a solution to resolve. Most importantly, I haven't given up.

As a final comment, I've also noticed that many myositis sufferers seem to develop other illnesses alongside the myositis. With me it was neutropenia.

A number seem to develop intolerance to certain foods etc. Maybe these develop as a consequence to the body system being down and therefore not able to deal well with certain foods; these then become like poison to the body. In my case it was wheat and recently gluten. Therefore, if not already done so, I would strongly suggest any myositis sufferer to get a food intolerance test to see if there is any food etc that the body has grown intolerant to. Most likely it will not cure you, but it may help.

My thanks goes to my wife Jackie for all her love, care and support over the years. I know this disease has been harder on her than it has on me.

Case Studies – Juvenile Dermatomyositis

Gareth	**JDM**
22 years old	

At twenty-one I was a strong, muscular, qualified fitness instructor who played hockey for a London national league club. Wanting yet further challenges I applied and have been accepted into the Police Force. A modern day miracle when you know that I contracted JDM when I was only four or five years old.

I can't remember everything, but my parents tell me it was difficult to get it diagnosed, as too few doctors were aware of it. My parents had to make a lot of fuss to get me into hospital for observation and tests to find the cause of my pain and power loss. It is due to them that I am in the position I am today, along with a few good doctors and physiotherapists.

My first memory of knowing that I was ill was when children, who I had always been better than, were beating me at judo. I remember being very upset and wondering where all my strength had gone. I do remember having problems at school due to mood swings which I now know are a symptom of this illness. Soon I was so weak that I had trouble climbing the stairs and used a wheelchair when I went out as I could not walk very far at all.

After being diagnosed at a local hospital I was started on a large dose of steroids to shock my system into working properly. After about a year I started making monthly visits to a London hospital where there were specialists who really understood my condition. We had to leave very early in the morning to go to London, arriving at the hospital in time for breakfast before the first appointment of the day (quite an adventure the first few times). The physiotherapists would work me hard and did a lot of strength resistance tests on me. This session usually ended with a timed sprint along the corridor before going on to see the specialists, but it took a long time to cure me and I had to go onto cyclosporin to help me to come off the steroids.

For the last year of going to London for physio, I was cured of the illness. I was ten years old. I remember that when they tested my strength I could push the lady physio across the floor on her chair! When I had to sprint down the corridor the physio would run with me and I remember leaving her behind with my speed. I think they realized that I was very much cured.

I was determined to be as fit and strong as any of the other kids, so I tried very hard at all my sporting activities, especially my chosen sport of hockey following in my father's footsteps. With his encouragement, I played a lot and quickly improved, achieving a position in the county team at thirteen and playing with them at all ages as I grew and developed, until finally captaining the team at under twenty one. I also played for the East of England team from the age of fifteen, selected from the seven counties in this group. I still represent the county of Essex in the men's team but am unlikely to be able to play regularly at the top level due to police shift patterns.

Update

I don't think about my time with JDM very much nowadays as I am totally cured and life is very full for me, but I do hope my story will be encouraging to others.

I have been a policeman for three years now and am enjoying the variety and experience it affords me. This year I received a commendation for restraining a man from jumping off a multi-storey car park. Could this be seen as another life saved by the doctors who treated me so well, I like to think so. Although I can't play my league hockey every Saturday because of the shift patterns of the job, there are other compensations. I play for the British Police and am captain of the Essex Police team. So 'Goodnight all' and just remember if you see and hear the Blue's & Two's, it could be me on another life saving mission! So just pull over and let me pass, Thanks!

Rex and Carole
Gareth's parents

JDM

Our son Gareth was about five when it all started. During the previous year he had had many of the childhood illnesses and had become very lethargic. He was diagnosed by a paediatrician at our local hospital as having sunburn when he developed a rash. He steadily worsened, often lying on the floor in a lot of pain, until his father decided to take positive action. Referral to our local hospital would take a long time so our intention was to take him straight to a London hospital as an outpatient.

When our GP realised our determination he spoke to a senior paediatrician who agreed to see Gareth before his next clinic. He was immediately admitted for observation and tests, to an otherwise empty children's ward! Fortunately for us, our local hospital had a new neurophysiology test machine and three days later they were able to give us a diagnosis of JDM and more importantly that there was a cure.

Gareth did not want to be different and was as determined as we were to beat this illness. Consequently, he took his medicine as prescribed and did all the exercises which his mum put him through!

Locally, we asked about a support group and were eventually put in touch with Les and Irene Oakley (Myositis Support Group). They knew our problems, our frustrations and our needs. They recommended that we should ask to be referred to the H Hospital in London as they specialise in these types of diseases, advice we are so grateful for! The type of physiotherapy prescribed by the specialists at the hospital was extremely important to his recovery.

Gareth started on prednisolone (steroids) daily, which was reduced at regular intervals. Cyclosporin was added to help wean Gareth off the prednisolone for 20 months and then he had cyclosporin by itself for 13 months.

We are members of a local church so Gareth was prayed for regularly and we believe God was on our side throughout.

Fast approaching 23 years old, our son now looks and is, a fine figure of a man with good prospects for a healthy and happy future.

Kim   **JDM**
17 years old

When I was diagnosed with juvenile dermatomyositis I was relieved. Someone finally believed what I had been saying for months. I thought the doctor would just give me some medication, I'd stay in the hospital for a few days and within two weeks I'd be back to the way I used to be. Was I wrong or what?!

My first symptoms were a constant ache everywhere and no painkiller would take even the edge off the pain. I had a red rash which covered my face – it was almost like a big butterfly. It was itchy and burnt. It was always a lot worse when I was tired or out in the sun. Over time my body became stiff and I was always drained of energy. Simple things became so much harder – walking, brushing my teeth, opening bottles. I went to see my GP most days and I was always off school. I had a few tests done, but when nothing showed up, people began to doubt my illness. It obviously never occurred to anyone that just maybe I was being tested for the wrong things. Most of the doctors I saw believed my problem was hormonal. I remember in particular one doctor literally throwing me and my mum out of his room, shouting that I was about to start my period and had to be rushed home! The other doctors believed my problem was psychological. They thought that I had trouble at school and that if people believed I was ill I could stay off. Now that I am older I believe that most doctors think that if an illness isn't easily found then it can't exist. How many people have to die before this misapprehension is changed?

Springtime came and things got much worse. I remember going shopping with my mum and I kept falling over – my legs just gave in! I was still at my GP's every day. I couldn't roll over in bed any more, have a wash or get dressed. I couldn't breath very well and I could hardly swallow. I was sent for blood tests and I couldn't even straighten my arm for the nurse to put the needle in.

It was a Thursday when I was diagnosed. My mum got me up early to see the doctor again. I remember going in to my nana's room where she dressed me in a brown T-shirt and a pair of black checked trousers. My mum brushed my hair. At the doctor's my mum carried me into the waiting room. I was given a chair as I kept falling when I stood.

Everyone stared at my red, cracked, bleeding face, all asking how my mother could have allowed me to become so sun burnt!

The GP didn't know what else to do for me. He said he had never seen anyone as bad as I was. He immediately sent me to the hospital. At 1.40pm I went into the consultant's room. He saw the rash, listened to my symptoms and he knew what was wrong with me.

He then did an examination and some tests and was shocked to see that I couldn't do the simplest of things that everyone takes for granted. I couldn't walk unless I was on my tip-toes and when he lifted me onto the floor I couldn't get up no matter how much I tried. In the words of my mother, I looked like a duck on ice!

I was admitted to hospital and given a strong steroid drip and pumped full of painkillers. The nurses kept trying to get me to eat something. I was really underweight but I didn't have the energy to even sit up while my mum fed me. By this time I couldn't get my arm to bend to put the food in my mouth. I don't remember much of the first day in hospital apart from sleeping all of the time and constantly being visited by doctors who had never heard of this disease before. I only remember being told that if I had waited and not gone to see the GP that day, I wouldn't have lived until Monday.

The next few months of my life was taken up by hospital visits. I saw a physio (called A) twice a week. I won't lie, I hated going. She forced me to do things that I really couldn't and sometimes I hated her for what she made me do. But looking back now, if she hadn't made me do those things, then I wouldn't be able to walk today. I also had hydrotherapy once a week. This was nowhere near as bad as I thought it would be. Then every Tuesday I went to see my doctor on the Children's Day Ward because it was much more comfortable there. There were a few nurses who worked there but one in particular, J, helped me the most. She always made me and my mum smile and was always really cheerful and friendly.

I had to have tests on my heart and lungs because the disease had taken such a hold on me. I had damage to my lungs which explained why I couldn't breath very well. My heart was fine – the disease hadn't harmed it. They only found a heart murmur.

September came and I tried to go to school for a day. I stayed for just under an hour before I had to come home. For the rest of year eight I never went to school. I had a home tutor who came for two hours a week. School work was hard. I couldn't write or hold a pen, so I was given a laptop but I never got the printer for it until two weeks ago – it was only three years too late!

If I went out, I went with my mum while she pushed me around in my wheelchair. The medication made me put on a lot of weight. I didn't look or feel like me anymore. I was put on cyclosporin too because the steroids were not working alone. Getting the dose right was tricky, sometimes I ended up in hospital because the dose was too high and I was overdosing.

From then onwards things slowly got better. I could swallow and feed myself again. When I got to year nine the illness seemed to die down a lot and I could very slowly start to come off the tablets. It took months but it happened. I was still in the wheelchair but everything seemed so much better. I had to start the long task of building my muscles up again. This was hard and tiring! At the very end of year nine I could go into school for an hour a day when I was well enough. I stopped the physio and hydro and saw the doctor less often.

Year ten came and I went back to school. I made loads of new friends and I was able to do most of my work, but some of the work was really hard, as I had missed so much. I still had a few bad times and I still went into hospital on the odd occasion. I eventually lost all of the weight and could do most of the things other people could.

In February of that year I met my boyfriend, Dan. Dan has helped me so much. He's helped me to do things I never thought I would be able to do. In that Spring I went away with some friends under the school's supervision. I went river walking, absailing and even climbed a waterfall! Not bad for a girl who was told she may never walk again!

In a few weeks' time I'll be seventeen. I still see the doctor every six months, I get tired and have a small amount of pain every now and then – but nothing is as bad as four years ago. I am waiting for my GCSE results and will be going to college. I can do all sorts of things that I never thought would be possible. I even have a job as a dance teacher for a drama group! I do ache afterwards but to me it's worth it.

For anyone reading this who has dermatomyositis, it's hard, we all know this but you WILL get through it. It gets so much better, but it takes time. You need to know your limits and don't push yourself too hard. That was always my biggest problem. I thought that I had missed out on so much that I didn't want to waste another second. I wanted to go out and do everything and I got so frustrated when I couldn't. But it puts you back when you push it and you feel like hell. Learn from my mistakes and don't do it.

I don't regret having the illness. It's changed me a lot and I believe I also got a lot out of it. I know more about life than my friends do and I've had so many experiences – not all good – but they have all helped me to grow as a person. Now I'm so much stronger than a lot of people I know. I'll fight for what I want and I don't give up easily. The biggest lesson I've learnt is not to let life pass you by – it's too short.

Since I won't get the opportunity again I'd like to thank a few people. First my family, I wouldn't have been strong enough without your support and love – thank you for everything you did.

My little sister Beth. I remember the times you pushed me around in the wheelchair and the times you came to physio with me, so you could learn the exercises then help me do them when we got home. I'll never forget. I'll love you forever girl.

To A – you made me walk again. You do a great job – thank you so much.

To Dr S – you saved my life. Thanks to you, no one would ever know that there was anything ever wrong with me. You're the very best at what you do. I'll never be able to thank you enough. Thank you.

And the most important person, I would never have been able to cope without her. My mum. You were there from the very first day and you never left my side. When times were bad you still kept strong and carried on for me. You never once let me down. You went way beyond the call of duty. You are the most amazing mother ever. Thank you for everything. I love you.

Update

Since I last wrote I have been to college, had to leave university and am currently holding down a full time job. After my GCSEs I decided to go onto college to do a course in Health, Social Care and Early Years with the hope of then going to university to do nursing. The first year of college was difficult as I was doing four A level courses and was a full time student. At that point in my life I found things increasingly difficult as my health was still not 100% and college was putting a huge strain on me. I was having to spend a lot of time off ill and this was affecting my work. After a few months I decided I could not continue with what college was doing to my health and so I dropped two subjects. This turned out to be the best thing that I could have done as I started to pick up and do well again. I started to really enjoy college and my course. My work was of a high standard and I met and made some amazing friends. I began to do all the things that everyone else did and for the first time in a long time I felt what I considered to be 'normal'. I went out with my friends all of the time, to the pub, the cinema, for meals, shopping and even concerts. Don't get me wrong, there were times when I was in a great deal of pain and was tired but with DM this is something you learn to live with but I decided a long time ago that DM would not dictate or control my life.

Once I left college I got a place on a nursing course at university, however, to get to the university I had to get three buses there and two trains home everyday as well as doing a full-time course nine to five everyday along with all the work which needed to be done. This killed me – to say the least! I had taken far too much on and my health began to become an issue once again. However, I am incredibly stubborn and because the nursing was something which I really wanted I kept going until I was so weak that I caught Hepatitis A. As a result of this, I was very ill for a long time and had to give up the nursing. Giving up university was an incredibly difficult decision but the Hep A taught me that although nursing was what I really wanted, you have to pick your battles more carefully. That's not to say I just gave up, maybe one day I'll go back to university and do the course and I'll be fine, but for now I'm happy with what I'm doing.

When I started to feel better I started to look for a job. I was lucky enough to find work as a Senior Nursery Nurse in a lovely nursery. Here I work in a baby room and look after children between the ages of 0-1 year. I love my job. I get to work with some lovely people and I feel very competent at what I do. So I guess I have been so lucky. I still have my bad days, but who doesn't? Yes, I still get pain and I get tired but nothing compared to what it once was. I have a great job, a hec-

tic social life and some of the best friends a person could ask for. But most importantly I have a fantastic family, who have been there with me every step of the way. In particular, my beautiful little sister.

I guess I have learnt that we will have some really hard times where the pain is so bad you wonder if it will ever stop. We will have times when things won't go the way we want them to but as I am writing this trying to remember the bad times, I can't. I remember the happy times where both mentally and physically I have felt strong. We should be so proud of our achievements however small they may seem to others and although it's hard, let the bad times fade.

Lynn (Kim's Mother)   JDM

In the autumn of 1996 my daughter Kim started to deteriorate. I noticed that she was coming home from school saying that she did not feel well. She was getting aches and pains all over and had constant pain in her head and neck. Kim had just started a new school and the doctors all thought that it was because she was not happy there, that she was getting the pains. She began to be sent home from school every few weeks with mainly stomach and chest pains and generally not feeling well. After the Christmas holidays when she returned to school in 1997, things were a lot worse. By this time I was walking her round to her friend's house every morning and the friend's mother would then drive them both to school. Kim could not carry her own bag because it gave her head and neck pain and she felt that she could not breathe when she was walking. All the way to her friend's house she would keep falling over because she said her legs kept giving in on her. I noticed little things, like she couldn't open bottles of pop I gave her with her packed lunch, or locks on her bag. When I told these things to one of my GP's, he said it was only stress or her age and to ignore it.

Things started to come to a head in April of that year when she was taken to hospital with stomach problems. When we got into hospital I noticed she had a very bright red rash on her face and neck. I did not know what it was and no one seemed too bothered about it.

She was put under the care of a doctor who saw her every month in his clinic. She had to keep a diary for him of all the times she was off school or felt ill. The diary was full of incidents of aches and pains and days off school. He told us that this record and the fact that she had a red face proved that she was going to start her periods. It got to the stage that I was sending her to school, only to be sent home ill again, within a few hours. We lived at the doctor's or the hospital but seemed to be getting nowhere. I was made to feel like a fussy mother with a spoilt, silly daughter who panicked about a bit of pain or a headache.

By the middle of July, Kim had been off school for a few weeks and was still getting no better. I decided that if it was in her head I would make her get up and get over it, so I made her walk her younger sister to school with me. We had to stand around for about half an hour as her sister was going on a school trip and I had promised to wave her off. The coach was late and all the time Kim kept complaining of pain in her legs and back. Her face was so red; it was cracked and bleeding. She looked awful. All the way home she kept tripping up and falling over. She went straight to bed as soon as we got home and stayed there for the rest of the day. The next morning she was very ill and I had to lift her out of bed. She could not dress herself, brush her hair, straighten her arms or even swallow, so I decided for the third time in a week I would take her back to the doctor's.

This time it was a GP who listened and he made arrangements for her to be seen at the hospital that day. As I sat in the waiting room at the hospital I just kept thinking how am I going to make the doctor listen to us and believe us. I was getting desperate as she was getting worse and worse all the time and no one was doing anything about it. We walked in and Dr S looked at Kim's face, then her knees, elbows and her knuckles. All these places had the same rash and we had not even noticed. You could not miss how bad her face was but we thought it was an allergy to something. He asked her lots of questions, then he made her sit on the floor and try to get up again. I was shocked to find that she could not do this, she just kept falling back down. He knew straight away what was wrong. We were told to sit back down and the doctor told us all that he could about the illness and how he hoped to treat it. I was so glad she was going to get help and yet afraid about what was going to happen to her. She had to stay in hospital and be put on a drip straight away.

As the days went on questions started to come into my head

but none of the nursing staff could answer them. Nobody knew anything about dermatomyositis. I knew that Dr S would have answered any questions I had, but every time I saw him Kim was there too and I did not want to ask my questions in front of her. I was sure she was going to die. I could not see how someone so ill, someone who could no longer dress herself, walk, brush her hair, feed herself or turn over in bed could get better. If they had said she had something like flu I would have known what to expect, but this was something I had never heard of.

One of the most frightening things to see was when she tried to feed herself, found it difficult to swallow and would then choke on her food. I just needed some information and to know what to expect. I found it difficult to talk to anyone about her illness at first, as I was afraid that if I did, I would start to cry and I didn't want to show any emotion in front of Kim. I tried to be happy and full of life when I was with her. I could not let her see that inside I felt like a train about to crash. On the outside everything looked fine but on the inside I felt panic and fear. I never left the hospital until she came home with me and on the last night before she came home, one of the nurses gave me a phone number for the Myositis Support Group.

I called this number as soon as I got home and asked all the questions I could think of. It felt great to speak to someone who had been through this and come out the other end. I felt much better afterwards and this was to be the first of many calls!

We used to go to the hospital four times a week for one thing or another and there were times when she seemed to be getting much worse. She had many stays in hospital and I always stayed with her. In a way this has been good for us, as I am so much closer to her now. She was always a bit of a tomboy and quite hard to get close to, but now we are very close.

I can still remember the times at physio when she used to be in so much pain. Sometimes she would lie on the floor and tears would be all over her face and I just wanted to pick her up and say you're never going back again, but without that she would not be as well as she is now. She spent a few years in a wheelchair and put on so much weight from the medication that even her school friends didn't recognise her. It would take forever to write about all the bad times Kim had and I could not put into words just how bad some of them were. But with time, things did start to get better and like you feel when you have a new baby, I felt proud of her when she started to do little things again, such as brush her own hair and eventually have a shower alone.

If an outsider looked at her today they would not believe that there was ever anything wrong with her. She is tall and very slim, has a boyfriend and does most things that she should be doing at her age. I am not trying to say that she does not get aches and pains and still finds some things difficult because that would be a lie. But she has been away with the school three times or more since she got better. Once to London, and the other times to Wales where she has done things like river walking. Not bad for a girl who used to be in a wheelchair.

Kim missed about three years of schooling as she was too ill to attend, but she has just sat her GCSE's and in a few days will get the results. To me it does not matter about the results because I could never be as proud of her as I am now. When I look at her I remember what she has been through and how brave she was as she fought to get better. I think I only ever saw her cry a handful of times. Most of the time she was just determined to get well and that is just what she has done.

Kim now teaches dancing to young children and teenagers and she loves it. By the time she gets home she can hardly walk, but she says it's worth it! Hopefully by the end of this week she will have a place in college. Back in the bad days I could never have hoped or dreamed that she would be like she is now. I really did not think she would get over it, but with a lot of fight and determination she is well again. She never moaned or asked 'why me?' She just got on with it and fought hard.

When you come so close to losing a child, life takes on a new look. Silly little things don't matter and there are very few situations which can't be sorted. I am very proud of both my daughters as little Beth lived her own kind of hell watching and helping Kim get better. When I was spending all the time with Kim she must have felt left out but in a strange way I think Kim's illness has made us all better people.

If I could change one thing, it would be to ask doctors to listen more – don't put everything down to stress and don't send people away feeling helpless. But no words can ever thank Dr. S enough.

On all the occasions that I have taken Kim to hospital or phoned up for help none of the nursing staff have ever heard of JDM. Once when I phoned the hospital to say she was having problems with her breathing, a senior nurse on hearing that Kim had JDM said, 'If she's got a skin problem, see your own doctor.'

I really feel strongly that myositis needs to be taught about more. I know it's rare but when you are going through hell, it's not very encouraging to be treated by people who don't know anything about it.

Su   **JDM**
30 years old
___

I was diagnosed with juvenile dermatomyositis in 1978 when I was six years old. Back then things were different. They knew little about the disease apart from the fact that it is very rare. Because of the rarity my mum wrote to newspapers and magazines trying to find someone in the same position as me. My mum received over 100 replies. Some from people with active illness or their kids who had it, but also from people who were in remission. I think this gave my family more hope knowing we weren't the only ones in the country that had to cope with this disease. Doctors had originally told my mum that there were only 3-4 people in the country that had it.

The one important person that kept me going throughout the early years was my mum. She fought for the best treatment for me. She ended up taking me to a doctor in Holland when doctors in Wales had near enough given up on me. They had left me on high doses of steroids and another drug and I couldn't reduce them without going 10 steps backwards. We didn't have the funds to go to Holland and without our knowledge our village raised the money for us. It was their kindness and generosity that enabled us to go.

In Holland I was put on a special diet consisting of high protein and phosphate and I had to drink four litres of fluid a day to flush my system of the steroids. After three months I was drug free with no ill effects. The treatment in Holland consisted of massage, reflexology and a special diet, but the most important thing was to work with the

Mind, Body and Soul as one. Some people might mock it, but it worked for me. Whilst I was there I was able to walk without difficulty, without being out of breath and I could also climb stairs which I was unable to do before I went.

I had a great time there. I went to a Dutch school and even learnt to speak Dutch fluently! I met some great people, some of whom I still keep in touch with. I learnt a lot about people, feelings and emotions. In a way I grew up very fast in Holland. I think growing up too quickly is a trait of young people with a chronic illness. I am still medication free to this day.

After Holland I was treated in a hospital in Berks. My consultant was a specialist in rheumatoid arthritis but also treated kids with JDM. I went to this hospital because even though my JDM was under control my calcifications had got worse. I was in a lot of pain and movement had worsened, something no one could have predicted. The main regime at this hospital was plenty of exercise, actually intense exercise, which helped me not to seize up even more. I would recommend every DM sufferer to keep moving. Again I met plenty of people who I still keep in touch with. From there I went to a college in Hampshire for my secondary school education. This is a college for physically disabled students.

This was the first school I had been to for physically disabled kids – scary – but I soon settled in. I suppose I learnt a lot about disability at that point. At first I had the same attitude as other people do about disabled people, not knowing how to react to someone in a wheelchair – even though I was in one myself!

The unknown is scary, until the known is approached without fear.

People are people regardless of how they get around or how they communicate.

The question is, what good has come out of having JDM.

- I've met many different and interesting people.
- If I hadn't been ill I wouldn't have had the experiences I had in Holland.
- I wouldn't have travelled to Taplow. I would probably still be living in Wales near my family.
- I have become independent. Apart from the places I've visited, I've tried to do what any able-bodied person would accomplish.

- I live in a house with my partner, Adrian, who has been a great help in my life. Without his push I wouldn't be driving a van as I do now!

Obviously things have been harder physically for me to reach certain goals but I've got there through people like Adrian, my mum and the rest of my family making sure that my world is as near 'normal' as possible. Whatever 'normal' is??????

With JDM/DM the key is not to give up hope. Life is worth living even though it gets tough now and again. My present condition is good. My DM is in remission but I still have some calcinosis and restricted movement. I use a wheelchair to get around as well as my van!

Medication free, my condition has stabilised and hasn't worsened in years. If anything I am improving slowly.

I am now 30 years old and try not to let the DM take over. I'm still under a local consultant in Alton and have also been back and forth to Holland for treatment over the years.

I just get on with my life.

Update

My condition still remains stable: no change, no pain. I am 33 years old now and currently a mature student. I decided to go back to full time education and take the challenge of doing a BA Honours degree. I am a first year student at Winchester School of Art, studying Fine Art Painting. I'm really enjoying it and it's great to meet so many creative people. It's also good that I'm not the only older student! I commute there everyday from Alton, in my van, which is great. I love the independence and would encourage anyone, whatever your condition, to learn to drive. If things get you down e.g. JDM or myositis, at least you can get away on your own, drive and have your own space (just to get away from it all!) Driving has given me more freedom and opens up new doors.

I have also joined an aqua therapy group, once a week, to help with exercise. I hadn't been having regular exercise from a physiotherapist for some time, as the authorities tell me they don't have the resources for someone like me; a chronic case! They tend to treat people who will improve. I still need to stay supple so I don't seize up completely. Surely movement and exercise is good for your mobility and well-being. I am in my wheelchair all day so it's great to be free of the chair in the water, move around freely and independently. Even though I can't swim, I have a life jacket on and it's great to be able to use my muscle power to its best ability. I love being able to move with the water taking my weight. Hydro-therapy is one of the best forms of therapy and can also be great fun!

Myositis is a horrible condition; just don't let it take over your life. Fight it by enjoying life to the full!

Del – Su's mum   JDM

In May 1978 Suzanne, at the age of six years, was diagnosed with juvenile dermatomyositis. The first thing we noticed was calcium coming out of her elbow and extreme weakness in her arms and legs. She was put on steroids, azathioprine and later chlorambucil. After a few years she was obviously making no progress and a doctor, who shall be nameless, was very blunt with us and said that nothing more could be done and that we should expect the worst.

That drove us to look elsewhere for another form of treatment.

We ended up going to Holland to see a specialist who believed in the body healing itself. We had nothing to lose and so for the next few years our lives changed dramatically as we travelled to and from Holland. She did improve for quite a while whilst receiving the treatment in Holland but then the calcinosis took over and her body was ravaged by deposits. She spent time in a London hospital.

At eleven, by then in a wheelchair, she went to a college for the disabled. The college did help her and she became more independent.

Suzanne now lives in a house with Adrian, her boyfriend (of the past 14 years), a parrot, a cockatiel and one rat! She drives a specially adapted van and drives down to Wales to see her family by herself – nothing stops her.

Even having had dermatomyositis, she's done so many things and met such wonderful people that she wouldn't have if she hadn't been ill. We'll never forget our friends in Holland who gave us their homes to stay in when we needed to. They are still our friends today.

As a family we are all very proud of her. When juvenile dermatomyositis was diagnosed in 1978 we thought it was a death sentence, but Suzanne has come out the other end a happier person.

Janelle   JDM
43 years old

I was diagnosed with JDM at the age of seven years. I do not remember a lot about that period of time, except for a few of the experiences that I endured. My earliest memory is going into hospital for my muscle biopsy. After waking up from the operation I discovered a huge plaster running down the side of my right leg from thigh to knee. To my horror I was made to get out of bed and walk around immediately. I was in pain and I remember thinking how cruel the nurses were. I now know the reasons why they did this, but at the time it was extremely difficult for me to comprehend.

I also remember my outpatients visits. Many students, who wanted to examine me and look at my face and hands, always surrounded me. Again I realise now that being such a rare condition, it was important for the students to see me. My consultant, Dr M, told us that at the time of my diagnosis in the mid sixties, he was a fairly mature man, (well he seemed ancient to me at the time!) he had seen about 20 cases of JDM world-wide!

My other memory is of the tests that I had to endure. Every visit to the hospital I had to have blood taken from my fingertips. Why from this particular place I do not know, I still don't to this day! This procedure was so painful and made my fingers so sore. I still have the scars now.

My parents always tried to make our visits to the hospital as pleasant as they could. We would travel from the Midlands by car and Dad would park on the outskirts of London. We would then get the Tube to the hospital for a morning appointment. Then we would always go to visit somewhere in the city, such as Madame Tussauds, the Post Office Tower etc. My sister and I were fortunate to have this opportunity to see so many interesting places. On the way home we would have a meal in a Chinese restaurant in Hendon, where over the years the staff got to know us quite well. My parents were not particularly well off financially at this time and I know that they had to make sacrifices to make these journeys, so I would like to say that I do appreciate what they did for me at this time.

My visits were gradually reduced over the years. As I got to my teenage years I became extremely self-conscious about the rash on my face. I was called awful names at school such as 'Spotty Dog' and as I was a sensitive person too, my feelings were hurt quite badly. I had some good girlfriends however and we all had many fun times.

By this time Dr M had retired and I was considered to be in remission. No more steroids now. The new consultant decided to try some cosmetic surgery on my face to try to reduce the rash, which was and still is quite severe.

Mr B attempted cryo-surgery to try to close off the capillaries beneath my skin. This was not successful, so he attempted a similar procedure using heat. No success again. I have since tried a laser technique to reduce the redness of the rash but again this only caused more scars.

By this time I had had enough of this surgery. I was referred to a cosmetic specialist for advice about camouflage makeup. I am so used to putting on my makeup every day now that my skin does not worry me as it did.

About the time of these cosmetic operations, I met Steve who is now my husband. I was about 17 years old. I remember coming home from London with a swollen scarred face and crying to my mum that he would turn and run a mile when he saw me looking so gross. Mum said to me, 'If he really cares about you it won't matter to him what you look like, it is the person underneath that is important.' She was right, he was totally unaffected by it all and we continued from there to have a great relationship for five years culminating in us getting engaged when I was 21 and marrying 18 months after that.

We have been married for 20 years now and I am very happy with my life. I have a career in Audiology at my local hospital where I am a part time Senior Audiologist. I have two healthy teenagers of 13 and 16 years. I lead an active healthy lifestyle, swimming, keeping fit and attending gym sessions at our local Health and Leisure Club. I have many lovely friends and supportive parents. My husband has a good job that means we enjoy a reasonable standard of living and enjoy lovely holidays.

I feel that I am very fortunate to be so well at the moment and I am doing my best to ensure that it stays this way.

The only negative part about this condition for me personally is the problem that I have with swallowing my food which seems to fluctuate with its severity and does affect me going out for a meal at times. I also get fed up with having to put makeup on all of the time before I can face the general public. I am not quite as sensitive as I was however. But as these are my only worries, I realise that there are many people far worse off than I am and I do have a lot to be thankful for.

Update

I am pleased to report that for the past 2 years, I have been fortunate to stay extremely well. The only medication I take now is Omeprazole for my hiatus hernia.

I continue to work in audiology and have increased my hours slightly, to help fund my eldest daughter who has now gone to university. We have enjoyed some great holidays as a family recently and I still regularly attend my Keep Fit classes. It is our Silver Wedding anniversary, my eldest daughter's 21st birthday and my son's 18th birthday in July and August 2006, so I am hoping that we can enjoy a lovely family holiday together again next year.

Fred and Joyce   **JDM**
Janelle's parents

Janelle was diagnosed as having JDM when she was seven years old. To some extent having a diagnosis was a relief, and to consult a doctor who understood the problems she was experiencing and who could probably treat her successfully relieved our worries, although we had not heard of the condition.

Looking back, I remember having problems keeping her hands, feet and nose warm during the winter months, from when she was only about 10 months old. This did not present too much concern at the time, as extra blankets, mitts and a bigger coal fire soon resolved the difficulty, but central heating in those early years would have been very welcome.

As a toddler, her hands and feet and nose became very blue during the cold weather, with very severe chilblains on her toes. The GP at the time checked her heart and suggested we should emigrate to a warmer climate!

Not a very practical proposal for us in retrospect!

Each subsequent year she seemed to suffer more during the winter months when the weather was cold. In particular, her fingers and toes became very blue with gangrenous patches developing on chilblains on her toes which took ages to heal. Gradually other symptoms began to appear. There were skin changes, a tightening and thinning, this had the effect of restricting her movements, which resulted in loss of balance and consequently she fell over fairly frequently. She tended to stay indoors more and she became an avid reader which had positive educational benefits. The rash on her face was particularly distressing and resulted in hurtful name-calling. She became very thin with some swollen joints, which gave the appearance of a developing arthritis, which is a familial condition.

The paediatrician decided to treat the symptoms as Raynaud's disease and the medication prescribed certainly helped with the susceptibility to the cold. A referral to a dermatologist and a further referral to Dr M at a London hospital resulted in an immediate diagnosis of JDM and treatment was started with prednisolone.

Janelle started to improve quite quickly and was soon able to enjoy a new bicycle, which she had craved, but previously had not had sufficient balance to ride.

As she got older, there were a variety of problems, but none so worrying as in the early years. These were balanced by the educational success she achieved, and by the lovely personality she was developing.

I became a very overprotective mother, especially during the primary school years when I defended her corner against the hurt caused by children and adults who did not realise how cruel they were being. Looking back, many of these incidents are quite amusing, but at the time, the support services, now available, were not in place.

The problems at school were generally quickly resolved by talking to teachers who were very understanding. She was allowed to stay in school at break times. Her peers, being told of her difficulties stopped the name-calling and she made life long friends with her classmates.

On one occasion I became very irritated with the 'nit' nurse who had isolated Janelle from her class, causing her great distress, presuming that she was infectious!

Physical education at her senior school caused another 'fight'. The PE teacher loathed to let Janelle make her own decisions about being excused, a note was required each time. Eventually Dr M came to the rescue and wrote a letter for her and thus she could choose her own activities during the lesson and avoid games such as hockey, even if she did 'skive off' at times!

We always made our appointments at the London hospital an exciting family day out, visiting places of interest around the consultation. The staff at the hospital were wonderful and took a very concerned personal interest in her case. Dr M seemed as pleased as we were when she passed the exam to go to the local grammar school.

The prednisolone was prescribed until Janelle was in her early teens and then she was weaned off the drug without too many problems. She continued to attend the hospital for research purposes and for attempts at cosmetic surgery until she was 21 years of age – but Janelle can continue the story herself.

In conclusion – although the early years were very distressing, we weathered the storm with the help and support from our Church, understanding relatives, friends and teachers. We are appreciative of all the medical staff who have been involved over the years and we thank them for their kindness and caring. Apologies to the younger sister who may have thought Janelle was getting more than her fair share of attention although we desperately tried to treat them equally.

Finally, we have a wonderful daughter who still experiences some health problems. But she has a lovely personality, a successful interesting job, a super husband and two healthy children.

Lindsey   JDM
21 years old

I was diagnosed with JDM when I was seven years old, after feeling unwell for quite a time. This diagnosis led to a more positive outlook for the future, as it had taken some time for a correct diagnosis to be made. Physiotherapy, steroids and support from my family and friends led me to being discharged completely when I was twelve years old.

I find that many things have helped in my recovery, such as the help and advice from health care workers e.g. Doctors, nurses and physiotherapists. I was prescribed steroids, naprosyn and hydroxychloroquine. I remember my mum used to hide my tablets in Weetabix, which made me want to heave! I hate Weetabix to this day!

My doctors, Dr S., Prof. B., Dr B-B. and Dr L. were essential in my recovery and all still have teddy bears named after them!

Part of my regular medication was cod liver oil, which I am sure helped to keep my joints more supple, even though it tasted disgusting!

I think the most important factor in decreasing pain in JDM is exercise. A physio programme was set up for me to do twice a day. My dad was chief physio at home and he set up an old bike on blocks so that I could pedal away whilst watching 'Neighbours!' I also enjoyed my swims in the hydrotherapy pool.

The support of my friends and family throughout this period was vital. I do not really remember much about being ill. Whether I was too ill or have blocked it out of my memory, I'm not sure.

I remember Mum, Dad and my two big sisters, Helen and Clare always being positive and trying to cheer me up. They provided round the clock care for me and treated me like a 'normal' child, no matter how ill I got.

The support of a good childminder, my family's wider circle of friends and my grandparents was also important. They could look after me when Mum and Dad were at work and my sisters at school. Also my friends at primary school and my friends now have been a big help in keeping me happy.

I believe that if you have been ill, you appreciate life more and my life now has more purpose. I would like to help others, the way those who were involved in my care helped me. I am just finishing my second year at the University of Greenwich doing a degree in Health and Learning Disabilities. I found that my own experiences led me to want to help children with physical and learning disabilities. I am thoroughly enjoying my course and have had the amazing experience of working with such children. I am also working part-time as a care assistant for the elderly.

In reflection, JDM is a severely painful and disabling condition and we must promote and try to raise more funds into researching the myositis conditions. But things do get better.

I am completely discharged, rarely suffer from aches and pains and scarring is minimal. It is important to keep a positive state of mind as well. The support of The Myositis Support Group has been a big help in raising friends' and family's awareness of the conditions. I urge those with myositis conditions to get in contact with them and especially to attend the AGM meetings.

And if you find that people stare at you when you are in a wheelchair, just stick your tongue out at them. I found it works a treat!

Update

Since writing my story for the book, things have changed slightly! I am living in Staffordshire, working as an unqualified social worker for an older person's team. It's something I really enjoy and I'm hoping to go back to university in the near future to do a Masters in Social Work which would open up many opportunities. Eventually I would like to work with children with special needs.

I have also become the Patient Representative for the JDM Registry and Repository Steering Committee. This entails a trip to the Institute of Child Health in London, a few times a year, to discuss research proposals etc. It's a very interesting day, especially considering how much research is now being done in comparison to when I had JDM many years ago. The people involved are fantastic and really want to make a difference to the lives of people with JDM. I also get to visit Oxford Street afterwards – always a bonus!

I continue to keep well, regardless of the odd flare up of calcinosis. All in all, life is treating me and my family well.

Susan and Patrick   **JDM**
Lindsey's parents

Lindsey first showed signs of JDM on a lovely family holiday on the Isle of Wight. Whilst there Lindsey developed a dry skin and eczema on her ears. When we got home our GP diagnosed infected eczema and prescribed antibiotics. After about a week she began to complain of pain and stiffness in her knees. They looked swollen and discoloured and our GP decided to try anti-inflammatory drugs. They only succeeded in making her feel sick and had no apparent beneficial effects.

Lindsey gradually became weaker and more unwell, becoming miserable and not wanting to do anything. She was going to her grand-

parents and child minder and was looked after by her dad in the afternoon, as school became more and more part time. The GP eventually
decided to refer Lindsey to a local paediatrician, but after several con-
sultations we were no further forward with a diagnosis. I looked up
every available medical book and always skimmed over DM as the
prognosis was so poor and I did not want to even consider that diagnosis. In the end, after trying different NSAIDs and aspirin and still her
condition deteriorating, we were referred to a rheumatology centre in
Birmingham. By this time Lindsey was losing her hair rapidly and had
become increasingly immobile.

Eventually, after waiting for an appointment, Lindsey was seen at
S.O. Hospital by three consultant rheumatologists who almost immediately gave us a diagnosis of JDM. This was confirmed a few days later
when she was admitted for tests and muscle and skin biopsies.
Following the confirmation we were sent home with steroids to treat
the condition and instructions for intensive physiotherapy to improve
the movement in her joints, which by this time had become fixed with
contractures. The therapist started to stretch her joints.

We had a holiday arranged, camping in the south of France and it
was agreed we could take her if we kept the sun off her fragile skin. We
went armed with high factor sun creams, a parasol for the wheelchair
and lots of light clothing to keep her covered. We had a tortuous journey and an eventful holiday, including a flood in the tent during a thun-
derstorm! But, Lindsey thankfully seemed a little stronger.

The diagnosis had come a year after the onset of symptoms and in this
time Lindsey became a very sick child who looked as if she would break
if you hugged her. However, once the steroids got to work and reduced
the inflammation, she began to improve. The encouragement of her
older sisters, her dad and the physiotherapist also helped enormously.

Hydroxychloroquine to improve the skin problems and hydrotherapy at the local special needs school allowed Lindsey to be back at
school full time and she began to get stronger and more mobile all the
time. Gradually we were able to leave the wheelchair at home and be
a 'proper' family again. Lindsey went from strength to strength, with
the odd setback. She took part in most school activities and learned to
play the flute successfully enough to be in the school orchestra. She
won the school music trophy when she left to go to secondary school.

Lindsey was very brave when she was ill. We, as a close knit family, worked together to make life more bearable for her and to get her better when she was so ill. I feel that we are probably closer for the experience we all shared in those bad days of JDM and we are all thankful she made the brilliant recovery she did. We are all proud of the fact that she is studying at the University of Greenwich to help people with physical and learning disabilities.

Leanne   JDM
15 years 11 months

When I was two and a half years old I began to find it hard to walk. My mum kept taking me to the doctors to be told that she was being over protective. My mum knew something was wrong and kept taking me back, until a trainee doctor noticed the symptoms of JDM.

Many doctors could not believe it when I had a blood test that showed I did have JDM. My doctor said I would miss loads of school and have many problems. My hospital had never had a child so young with the illness. I was put on prednisolone.

I am now 15 and am leaving school in a couple of weeks. I have been at school nearly every day for the last 12 years – only having time off for hospital appointments.

I've had many doctors and they're usually amazed when they find out what I can do! I used to do championship swimming, skipping and gymnastics, but now I do break dancing! When I go to the hospital they always ask me to do some moves!

Two years ago I was taken off prednisolone and put on to azathioprine. Because of my illness I am very small. I look about 12, which I don't mind because I get in at child rate everywhere!

My mum has helped me a lot. She takes me to hospital and has always helped and encouraged me in whatever I want to do.

I also go to a performing art school at weekends where I dance, sing and act. I did a film with Patrick Stewart and Richard E. Grant called 'A Christmas Carol.' I've also been in 'The Bill'. I love acting the most.

My friends are really nice. On days when I felt a bit tired they were always there to carry my bag or help me with little things. At dancing class my friends can't believe that I have an illness. I used to hear, 'Oh my nan has that!'

I don't let having JDM control me. In my head I think I can do anything I want, so I do!

I get a few aches and pains but they're nothing compared to having fun!

When I leave school I'm going to college. I want to do art and acting when I'm older.

I went to the doctor last week and was told that there were no traces of JDM in my blood. It has taken 13 years but at the moment I'm OK. Hopefully it will stay that way. I don't mind having JDM because it has made me what I am today.

By the way, when you have pains, heated bean bags are the best thing. Put them where you hurt and they take the pain away.

Never let anyone tell you, you can't do something because it's not true and I have proved it.

Today I can walk and dance!

Update

Things have really changed. I became allergic to azathioprine which made all my hair fall out. I was put back on steroids for a course of two weeks after another flare up. But I have been free of medication for the illness for nearly three years and it feels brilliant. I always think about my childhood when I was sometimes too weak to walk or stand. Well, now I'm driving, am a youth worker and dance teacher (teaching 6 - 30+ yr olds). It's keeping me very busy. I have danced in Paris and all the famous land marks like Her Majesty's Theatre, Saddlers Wells and the Royal Albert Hall. I'm still doing my acting and now music videos.

Still no-one believes my age. Growing up I hated looking young and being short, due to the steroids. But now, it's actually working to my advantage. I get more parts and jobs in the industry.

My family and boyfriend still help me when I have my low days of feeling tired and weak but it usually goes within two days (all thanks to the heated bean bag: nothing can beat that).

I go to the hospital regularly for checkups. On my last visit I was told I only need to come back twice a year, which is good news.

It feels like I'm finally just me. I used to always tell people I had

JDM, because I was scared of them hugging me too hard etc: now I find it doesn't even enter my head. I have scarring on my face from the illness. That's the only thing I find hard to deal with.

I'm now helping people to turn their lives around and build positive futures and attitudes. I'm hoping to work in the hospital that has helped me all my life.

Kate   JDM
20 years old

I was diagnosed with JDM when I was two and a half. My story is about the most positive one you will hear, I think! Yes, there were many down sides, but there were certainly enough up sides!

After a long time of struggling to find out what was wrong with me, we were sent a letter from my aunt with an advert for a hospital in London that she had come across by chance. She wanted to know if it would be any good sending me there. I was duly given an appointment (if it had been any later I wouldn't be here to tell the tale!) and diagnosed. I was treated with a cocktail of drugs, steroids, anti-inflammatories etc. You name it – I've taken it! Eventually, when I was about ten, they hit upon cyclosporin – a drug normally given to transplant patients to stop them rejecting their new organs. It worked. To cut a long story short, here I am, ten years on, completely free of the disease. OK, so I haven't mentioned the details, the bad bits, but as we all know, there are enough of those to go on about forever! What I remember most were all the great, and I do mean great things, which happened to me in the duration of the disease.

The most important factor in coping with the disease was the support of my wonderful family. We are all so close, and without them I would have lost hope long ago. I really feel that the disease brought us closer together, cemented our bond. Even though I suffered from the disease all through my childhood, I can remember that childhood being the best time of my life. My parents didn't let the fact that I was ill stop me from doing anything a normal kid does. The county council wanted to send me to a 'special school' for the disabled, but my parents were having none of it. They fought tooth and nail to have me sent to the local primary, and the council finally relented. There I had a care assistant, who used to give me physiotherapy. Although I felt different from the other pupils, I had a friend in Mrs. T (the carer), besides which she used to spoil me rotten!

Visits to the hospital were made fun – we used to go on the train, which in itself was exciting, then afterwards we would visit London, taking in the sites. We went to Madame Tussauds, the Museum of Moving Image, the Natural History Museum; the list goes on!

I must have been in the local papers five or six times within a space of five years. It was through this coverage that the local fire station and one fireman in particular, JM, heard about the disease. The station organised a sponsored cycle ride from Bridgewater to our twin town of La Ciotat, in France, to raise money for research into the disease. There was much media coverage, and when they came back from successfully completing the ride there was a big party to celebrate! The station also made me an honorary fireperson, which meant that I was invited to all their parades and 'do's'. They even came to pick me up for these events in a fire engine! As you can imagine, it was all very exciting for someone my age (I was about four or five at the time).

Then came the most exciting thing that has happened in my life to date. When I was about eight, JM, by now a family friend, nominated me for a 'Children of Courage' award, a scheme run by Esther Rantzen. They kept this a complete surprise from me, telling me that I was going up to Heathrow Airport for the day for a 'party'. My mum and I were taken by a fire van to the Hotel Sheridan, near Heathrow, where it was all taking place (we were very late, the firemen having had to stop and assist someone who had broken down. We then shot through traffic on the hard shoulder with the sirens going!) It was then that I found out I was going to travel on Concorde! We flew to the Bay of Biscay and back in under an hour and a half, and were visited on the plane by Father Christmas! It was the most fantastic experience. After arriving back at the airport, we were given lots of Christmas presents, and had the chance to meet Roy Castle. I was almost thankful to the disease on that day, for letting me have the chance to do what my friends back at school could only dream about.

When I was nine, I went on a pilgrimage to Lourdes in France. Again, it was a fantastic experience. Brought up a Catholic, there were lots of masses and services, where people, healthy or ill, could all come together and support each other, and talk about their experiences. I can only describe it as a very magical, spiritual experience. I recommend it to any sufferer, religious or not. One thing it taught me is that there are always people worse off than you are, and that you should never lose hope. I think that hope is the most important weapon we have in fighting our illnesses – lose that and you have nothing.

So, that is my story, along with countless other good things that have happened throughout the course of my disease. It is so important to realise that there are others out there who are in the same boat as you, so don't lose hope, you can beat this thing! And if you need to talk, then talk. Whether it is with a friend, relative, your doctor or whoever, it helps. Sometimes when you let your feelings out instead of bottling them up, things just don't seem quite so bad any more. And trust your doctors – they know what they're doing!

Update

I have been symptom free of JDM since writing my first story. Quite ironically, I am back on prednisolone as I have recently been diagnosed with Crohn's disease. I am slowly but surely on the mend.

4

Remission

Sherlock Holmes, we need you now!

by Richard Gay

Background

Clearly the most intriguing, perplexing and unresolved question for all myositis patients, especially dermatomyositis (DM) and polymyositis (PM) patients, is the issue of remission, how often it occurs and what makes it happen. One beautiful young woman who had just been diagnosed with PM came to our support group and asked with tears in her eyes, "What is going to happen to me? Will I ever dance again?" I wanted to give her a hug and a magic recipe for restoring her health: just do the following things and you will be well again. Alas, I could not give her any specific recommendation, or even predict her outcome with any certainty. Remission of myositis is a riddle befitting the most classic opera plot.

For our purposes here let us define remission as the absence of disease symptoms (muscle weakness, pain, skin rash, etc.) accompanied by normal diagnostic tests such as blood tests, electromyogram, magnetic resonance imaging, biopsies, etc. This is consistent with the common working definition used by autoimmune specialists at the US National Institutes of Health, and is a logical definition. From a practical viewpoint it may be an extreme definition because the word "inactive" is just as desirable because an inactive illness means we are over the worse aspects of the disease, but may still carry some out of range blood tests or symptoms as a carry-over from fighting the disease. In fact, DM, especially juvenile DM (JDM) is thought to have three characteristic forms: one in which only one very active period is followed by no flares or disease activity (ie, remission); a second form in which a cycle of inactive and active periods (called a flare) occur; and third, a continuously active disease which seems to never subside. The myopathies are never considered "cured" because by their nature, they are auto-immune, and one cannot conclude completely that the memory of the disease has been removed from our immune system, only to find it re-awakened by some future event. Consider that in the 1950's and 1960's almost everyone was inoculated for smallpox virus. In the interim time period the smallpox virus was eradicated, and yet health experts could not say if the people who were inoculated still carried immunity to the disease in the face of a potential terrorist release of the virus. Of course no one wanted to volunteer to test the hypothesis that their immunity had worn off with time! Once activated our immune system carries the memory of specific antigens, ready to produce new antibodies at any time. Thus even someone in remission begins with an inactive disease period of unknown duration, perhaps tempered with the hope that "permanent" remission could be achieved.

We can speculate that there should be adequate long-term health records available to clarify the statistics of incidence of occurrence for remission and active-inactive disease. Unfortunately this has not been clarified and may not be possible. For example, we can assume that the incidence rate of JDM has been constant for the last fifty years at about 3 to 5 per million per year. Prior to 1950 or so, synthetic cortisone (commonly available as prednisone) was not available and the mortality rate from JDM was very high. Prednisone was the miracle medication that saved the life of JDM kids and many others with auto-immune diseases, and the discoverer of prednisone quite appropriately received the Nobel Prize. We can make some rough estimates of how many JDM kids should be alive today in the United States if for example, one-third of them went into long-term remission. The number, just from the whole decade of the 1960's, comes out to be about 1500 to 2000 people. No studies have been done to find and track these kids, now adults in their 40's and 50's, and the number I am familiar with personally is much less than 10! Are the rest in remission and out playing golf? I don't know. My JDM is considered inactive but not in remission by our definition because my CPK is still slightly elevated. This could be sign of disease activity, or it could be muscle scarring from the time the disease was active. This lack of a working data base is compounded because the diagnosis of JDM, DM or PM may be incorrect. There are other diseases with similar symptoms to these autoimmune myopathies that could be incorrectly labeled as DM. If a treatment worked for them, they would be called in remission, but that treatment would not work for other DM patients. For example, some myopathies are caused by infections, not an autoimmune response. There are anecdotal reports of individuals who used long-term antibiotic treatment for DM and are now symptom and medication free. However, I know of two women with DM who used antibiotic therapy for over a year with absolutely no improvement. Antibiotic therapy for DM and PM is controversial and unresolved. For inclusion body myositis (IBM) patients there is no record of successful remission, and there is no successful treatment to alleviate the symptoms.

In addition, there are many patients who have autoimmune disease overlap. The myopathies are only one of many diseases that are autoimmune in cause. For example, rheumatoid arthritis, lupus, and scleroderma are autoimmune diseases. There is overlap in the symptoms and the basic treatment can be identical. One autoimmune illness may respond to treatment while the other does not. Thus it is very difficult to compile statistics in the long term for how many myositis patients have gone into remission. We do know that many kids with JDM do go into remission and are able to completely stop taking medications. Specific statistics for all myositis patients are not available in the literature, but generally about one third have a good outcome (inactive illness with little or no continuing medication), one-third control the illness with continuing medication, and one-third see a continuing decline in health even with aggressive medication.

Strategies Which Improve the Probability of Remission
The master detective Sherlock Holmes would be baffled by the mix of evidence making remission seem both at hand and out of reach. In our Los Angeles myositis support group I know of two young adult women who had PM and went into remission. The young woman I described

earlier is able to dance again. Yet upon questioning them, neither one could tell me of any specific action they took which caused their remission to occur. In an effort to learn something from others good fortune, we are forced to try to draw conclusions on the basis of individual stories from patients in remission or inactive DM and PM with wide-ranging backgrounds just searching for consistent, common factors. My recommendations are based on this and my forty years experience with the disease. We are not just corks bobbing up and down at the whims of the ocean waves, hoping that the right wave will push us into the bay of remission. We can identify an optimum strategy, which if implemented, positions us for remission.

1) Correct Diagnosis and Aggressive Therapy

In Renaissance times casting out demons was an art used to treat many illnesses. However, a demon could not be "cast out" until the correct name of the demon was known. Doctors took considerable time and made a very serious effort to correctly identify the demon. Although we tend to smugly think of ourselves as modern and much more knowledgeable than exorcists of demons, we must give our ancestors credit for recognizing that you must have the correct diagnosis (ie, know the correct name of the demon) to prescribe the correct treatment. We have much better diagnostic tools today, but an incorrect diagnosis can delay therapy at a critical time. Because myositis can be severe in the first few weeks, the correct diagnosis is a must and it should be followed immediately with aggressive therapy.

In 1964 the only treatment for JDM was prednisone. My JDM was diagnosed immediately when I saw my local doctor and I started on 30 mg/day of prednisone (about 0.5 mg/kg). I continued on that level for many years. My muscle strength returned to about 60% within a few weeks, but within a year I lost so much calcium from my back that I had to wear a back brace for five years. In the 1960's there were no effective medications to fight osteoporosis. In 1970 I started taking methotrexate and the prednisone dose was lowered. I was fortunate to see a leading rheumatologist, Dr Carl Pearson, at UCLA, who was an expert in myositis. Today the treatment is the same, prednisone, or a variation of prednisone, but the accepted strategy is to begin more aggressively, with about 1 to 2 mg/kg of body weight for the initial few weeks of treatment. The strategy is to hit the immune system very hard to stop the response. The prednisone dose is tapered off over the months following this treatment. This approach has been successful in achieving remission for many patients, especially those with JDM and PM.

2) Time

When I was first diagnosed with JDM in 1964 my doctor told me and my father that he expected the disease to "burn itself out" within two years. This was over 40 years ago. It actually took 17 years before I was able to stop taking prednisone. My skin rash and itching was a severe problem for 14 of those years. Time is a subtle but definite ally in fighting DM. One could say this is a waiting game. Given sufficient time it can burn itself out; that is, our immune response will taper off. However, we have to remain vigilant in controlling the long-term side effects of the medications such as osteoporosis, weight gain, cataracts, stomach ulcers, mood swings, liver upsets, etc. and the detrimental effects of the myositis, such as calcinosis, muscle wasting, contractures, injuries from falling, etc. Time is on our side though because it provides the opportunity for the disease to become inactive.

3) Treatment Protocol

When prednisone alone is not effective in controlling myositis, other treatments and medications are used to supplement the prednisone. This could include methotrexate, immuran, cellcept, intravenous immunoglobulin, etc. The exact combination varies from person to person, but the goal is to lower the prednisone dose while also controlling the illness. In addition, the side effects of prednisone can be mitigated by lowering the prednisone dose while using another medication to supplement it. Prednisone also leads to osteoporosis and recurrent infections, especially at the location of calcium deposits. In my case my doctor prescribed vitamin D supplements (50,000 units once a week) so that no new calcium deposits formed. The strategy is to control the disease and the side effects so that the situation becomes stable. Once stabilized, the combination of treatments can be lowered as the activity of the illness decreases. I monitored my strength as the prednisone was lowered by my ability to maintain a standard exercise program. I used muscle strength as a measure of DM activity, not blood test results.

4) Exercise

There was no data or information available to me in 1964 to provide a guide in fighting JDM. It made sense that the best approach to fighting a muscle wasting disease was exercise and that is the approach I have taken since then. Today there are many controlled studies which demonstrate that a consistent exercise program is important for maintaining strength and slowing the muscle wasting for myositis patients. Information on structuring an exercise program is available from many sources and is readily adaptable to the individual with myositis. In my experience, the important factor is to maintain the exercise program consistently. This requires internal discipline and is not negotiable. The patient with myositis does not have the luxury of being a couch potato. The case stories of people with myositis who did not achieve remission with the first aggressive dose of prednisone consistently show that exercise was a dominant factor in improving their health.

5) Emotional Health

I have seen and heard from others in our support group that they are depressed and taking medications for their depression. I have never had any serious depression even though my JDM was very serious. Depression seems to affect adults much more than kids with JDM, perhaps because adults seem to have unwarranted expectations of nothing going wrong with their health. My approach was to always systematically fight the disease and this requires being emotionally strong and healthy. There are many useful techniques to maintain good emotional health. For example, surround yourself with loving people, your family and neighbours, who are reliable, honest, good-natured and willing to assist you when needed. Walk away from people and family situations that are emotionally unhealthy. A household pet, such as a dog or cat, has a powerful positive emotional effect. When I was young with JDM my pet dog was an extremely loyal, loving fox terrier. Now I have three very loving cats. There exist large libraries of songs and brilliant music from the masters which is encouraging and inspirational. These composers have left this music precisely for our well-being. Take advantage of all of these aspects of your life. In order to fight the illness for the long term (recall time is our ally) good emotional health is a must.

6) Spiritual Health

One concept of who we are is a set of three concentric circles, somewhat like the target of a dart board or an archery match. The outer circle represents our physical body; the next inner circle is our emotional person, and the center circle is our spirit. If our spirit is alive, the remaining emotional and physical body can be carried by the strength of our spirit in the center. If your spirit is atrophied or even dead, we will not be able to keep ourselves going. Myositis is devastating because we have to maintain our spirit for a very long time. Little problems slowly add up. When I had my first electromyogram (EMG) test in 1964, I was 13 years old and I thought I was pretty tough. During an EMG a needle is inserted in the muscle and slowly moved around while the electrical signal is monitored by the operator. In my test the needle was pushed into my shoulder many times. It hurt each time but I didn't start crying until this had been done many, many times. I wasn't able to hold back. The same effect happens to our spirit. Repeated small incidents in our lives due to problems caused by the myositis will destroy our spirit. I have seen members of our support group begin an exercise program or diet but they lack the spirit to continue because it is no longer easy or glamorous. We do not match the ideal person constantly presented by Madison Avenue advertisers. Our self-esteem takes a big hit due to the side effects of prednisone and the myositis itself. Our spirit requires nurturing and strengthening to continue our exercise and diet with a pleasant attitude. We do not need to "re-invent" the wheel here. I found classical Judeo-Christian teaching to be extremely sustaining and life-giving during all the time I have had DM. The prophet Jeremiah (17:7-8) tells us "Blessed is the man who trusts in the Lord, whose hope is the Lord. He is like a tree planted beside the waters that stretches out its roots to the stream; It fears not the heat when it comes, its leaves stay green; In the year of drought it shows no distress, but still bears fruit." Spiritual health is vital; to stay on the path to remission we need a spirit that is alive.

7) Nutrition and Weight

Controlled studies have found that there is no specific diet that is beneficial or harmful to patients with arthritis. It would be logical to expect that myositis also is not affected by diet. My own experience is that specific diet is not critical, but I am underweight and I can eat a lot without gaining weight. However, prednisone increases appetite and is notorious for creating overweight patients. This extra weight is a big detriment for patients to carry with weakened muscles. Healthy people must eat properly to maintain their strength and myositis patients are no different. The weight has to be controlled.

8) Vitamins and Supplements

There is a lot of advertising for many different vitamins and supplements. A good vitamin supplement is useful for a healthy diet. However, I have tried many of the specialized supplements such as aloe vera, l-carnitine, Coenzyme Q-10, glucosamine-chondroitin, creatine and others and found none of them had a significant effect. One of our support group members has been using specialized oriental herbs for over a year with no benefit. These vitamins and supplements get a lot of publicity but have only a small effect.

9) Living Accommodations

There are many changes we can make to our living conditions which greatly simplify and make life easier for ourselves. For example, if you are having trouble climbing stairs, move to a one-story building, or only use the bottom floor of your house. Take the stairs out of your life. Buy three or four pairs of reachers to pick items up from the floor so you don't have to go down on your knees to pick things up. With myositis we drop small items all the time. Store the kitchen items you use most often at waist level to make it easier to reach them. Make your house safe from falling by removing small throw rugs and other items that can cause a fall. Have a cell phone readily available for calling friends in an emergency and be sure they have a key to your house. Change the chairs and other furniture items in your house to be easier to get up. Get a handicap licence for your car to park closer to stores. Have friends go shopping with you and buy enough for one or two weeks at a time to minimize the shopping trips. Magazines for muscular dystrophy and similar illnesses have countless recommendations to make life easier.

10) Keeping Busy
People who volunteer to help others have a purpose in life and fulfillment from the gratitude of the recipient. Most of us with myositis are capable of getting around and doing many things. If we can no longer work, we can use our time to help others or improve ourselves by participating in clubs and other organizations. It is important to have a reason to live and be needed by others.

All of the above factors are important for moving towards remission though none of them are unusual in comparison to what is needed for anyone to live a healthy life. I know of some myositis patients who simply take their medications and treatments and wait for something good to happen. Others actively take charge of their recovery and move themselves into a much healthier situation even if not full remission. In every instance it came down to the discipline and determination of the individual to make a plan and stay with it.

Richard Gay is the co-leader of the myositis support group in Los Angeles, California. He was diagnosed with juvenile dermatomyositis in 1964 at 13 years old. He was on prednisone for 17 years and was one of the original patients in 1970 to use methotrexate as a supplemental medication. He has personally experienced many of the side effects of myositis and prednisone: calcinosis, muscle contracture, severe skin rash and itching, growth inhibition, stomach ulcers, lipodystrophy, osteoporosis, and very limited muscle strength. He holds a PhD in Engineering from UCLA and was a technical staff member and manager for over twenty years in a chemistry research group for a large aerospace company. He is now retired and authors a bi-monthly newsletter for the Los Angeles support group.

Remission Case Studies

Liesl   **DM**
37 years old. Diagnosed aged 28.

Antibiotic Protocol

I was diagnosed with DM in September 1996. I began having symptoms – first a rash that would come and go, on my face and chest. It was light pink and a little itchy. It was like mild sunburn. This took place about 4-6 weeks after my second child's birth (June 1996). I had also received a rubella vaccine following his birth.

I was first told I had polymorphus light eruption – sun sensitivity. This didn't make sense to me since I am half Filipino and tan very easily. My Nurse Practitioner ordered some tests and after a week or two I got news that my ANA had come back positive. She suspected Lupus. I was seen by another doc at my General Practice office. By this time I was having muscle weakness. I had great difficulty rising from a chair, brushing my hair or teeth was torturous – my arms would burn after just a minute. My hands had a rash on them too. This doctor told me that I was probably carrying my 2 month old baby too much (causing the muscle pain and weakness) and I had eczema on my hands – probably from dishwashing. I stopped shy of calling him an idiot. He said the next step would be to see a rheumatologist – he gave me a referral to one who could see me in 6 weeks… I told the rheumy's office I couldn't wait that long – but they said the GP said it was okay for me to wait 6 weeks. I found another rheumatologist who saw me within a couple of days… he took one look at my hands and said he didn't think I had Lupus… he said he thought I had dermatomyositis. That was the first time I had heard that word.

He started me on 20mg of prednisone (this is low; normally he said it would have been 60mg but he didn't want to jeopardize the muscle biopsy he had ordered). The muscle biopsy was conclusive for DM… and the 20 mg of prednisone helped me to feel fine again. My CPK at the time was 983.

At first, after I was put on prednisone, this seemed to make me feel better. I remember thinking, "Oh, this is great – I feel fine, I am well – hallelujah!!" Little did I know that it would become a vicious cycle…

With each flare I would go up on the prednisone. As my symptoms diminished because my immune system was suppressed I would slowly decrease until the next flare and start again. Along with the prednisone came many undesirable side effects... moon face, weight gain, thinning hair on my head, hair growth where I didn't want it, hump on my back, thin skin, osteopenia... it was the lesser of 2 evils.

In 1998 I was able to travel for a month in Europe with my husband. I was on 5mg of prednisone at the time and was able to walk and hike and sightsee in France, England, Ireland, Italy and Austria.

I have also tried Plaquenil but I had an allergic reaction – hives all over me. I then tried Chinese Herbs and changed my diet according to a Naturopathic doctor... after 6 weeks I had a really bad flare with my skin rash resembling a second degree burn. It was so painful I could barely move. I remember going to the drugstore and barely being able to drive my car the 2 block distance. I bought Dermaplast – a topical anesthetic spray to numb my chest that was so raw and open.

At this time I found out about antibiotic therapy. I had read a book and done research online as well as corresponded with others who had used or were using the antibiotic protocol (AP). At my appointment with my rheumatologist he said he wanted me to go on methotrexate. I brought my info on AP – the book, the protocol, etc. He said it was not proven by double blind placebo testing and he didn't buy it. He said if it were him he would do MTX (methotrexate). However, he prescribed minocycline for me – to let me try AP for 6 months. I followed the protocol of 200mg Mondays, Wednesdays and Fridays – taken 100 in the morning and 100 in the evening. When I went back to see him I was taking a half mg of prednisone (cracking my 1mg tablets in half... I was just paranoid because I had never been off it before!)... he said I could stop taking the prednisone and had to wonder if it was the minocycline that was helping! I was medication and symptom free until the birth of my daughter in April 2001. In May 2001 my CPK was 2000... I went to my new GP who knew nothing of DM or AP (my rheumy had quit practicing medicine to make furniture)... he asked me lots of questions and he agreed to treat me with antibiotics... erythromycin would be safe for me to take while breastfeeding. Taking 250mg of erythromycin 2x daily, in 8 weeks my CPK was normal. I also took acidophilus daily to keep from getting yeast infections. I stayed on the antibiotics and gradually weaned down and then off. I've been medication and symptom free now for about 4 years.

Having DM when it is flaring is so difficult. I was only 28 when diagnosed and I had a four year old and a newborn. Prednisone gave me mood swings and I was very short tempered – which is not like 'me'. I had a lot of anxiety when I tapered the medications, wondering always if going too low would mean another flare. I never weaned/tapered unless my CPK was normal and I felt 'well'. I always went cautiously slow with tapering.

This time around it has been 4 years... I feel great, absolutely fine. I have a slight amount of residual weakness – I think due to permanent muscle damage...but it doesn't keep me from doing anything I want. I learned to snowboard a couple of years ago. I feel strong; have lots of energy (never nap!). I care for my 3 kids, dog, cat, 2 hermit crabs, husband, house, 5 rentals, teach religious education, work from home part–time, volunteer at the schools... you name it!

Mark   **DM**
40 years old. Diagnosed aged 31.

Recipe for Health with DM - Spring 2003

You and I have something in common. Either we, or someone we care about, is afflicted with a little known or researched family of diseases. We are unique. In the seven years I have had dermatomyositis I have never met, face to face, another person who shares my disease. I do better than most people with this illness. If you are reading this, it is probably because you want to know why and how. I am pleased to share this with you.

I would like to start by giving you a history of my battle with dermatomyositis so you may know my perspective and motivations. I feel that attitude and eating are most of the battle. The rest is a combination of controlled rest, intelligent and appropriate exercise and doctor's orders. However, I must have all these elements to succeed. I cultivated my attitude from lessons learned from my parents and life.

In early February 1996, I was diagnosed with dermatomyositis at 31 years of age. I had the classic symptoms of proximal weakness, tell-tale rash and sheer exhaustion. My lab work was basically unremarkable except for the EMG. The disease onset rate for me was particularly fast as I went from rollerblading 10 miles at a fast pace to barely lifting my head off a pillow in about three weeks. At one point I needed my father to help me climb steps. Initially, I was put on high dose prednisone daily and Imuran. My body did not tolerate the Imuran and we made the switch to methotrexate. I also did a 6 month IVIG regimen with great success. I slowly improved, tapered my medication and went back to work as an on-demand charter pilot, after six months. In October 1998, I earned a job with a major airline and my life improved dramatically as I was able to control my rest and diet better on a more predictable schedule.

I was also able to begin training in earnest for a goal I had set while I was very ill. My adventurous 7th grade English teacher, Diane Veneklassen, had swum the cold 4.1 mile Straights of Mackinaw some years earlier. If I could do that, then I was no longer a victim of a disease, I was the owner of one. My first swim in the pool was difficult. I struggled to do a dozen laps or so with lots of rest between each. A few days later I went a little farther. Eventually, I was able to plan a flexible schedule of swimming, biking and light weights, adding in days of rest when needed and reducing my planned training events as needed to accommodate the 'bad days' we all have with these illnesses. On August 13th 1999 at 6:50 in the morning I dived into the water at the southwest side of the Straights with my trusted friend Roger, at my side in his kayak. One hour and forty six minutes later I struggled out of the cold water and onto the rocks of the other side. As I sat crying on the cold rocks I knew I was no longer the victim of a terrible disease but I did not own it either. The truth was I had owned it for months as I trained and participated in endurance sporting events leading up to my swim. I did not want to own it. I wanted to be a partner with it. Had it not been for dermatomyositis I would never have known the feeling I had earned there on those rocks. I would rather not be ill, but, since I had no choice, DM and I were going to be partners. Later that fall, I completed the Ice Man, a 26 mile mountain bike race in northern Michigan in late November.

My next goal was to be med free. I reasoned that I had to back off my exercise regimen to do that. Boy was I wrong. Two things happened when I reduced my exercise. One is I lost my mindset that partnered me with DM. The second was an extension of the first......I stopped eating correctly. I was not training and therefore did not feel the same motivation to eat well all the time. In November of 2000, these two events would have disastrous effects as I became the victim (again) of a vicious flare up that had me rolling to get out of bed, exhausted 24/7 and unable to work. I had finished my year long taper off all meds just six weeks prior. I spent 3 months off work while I waited for prednisone and Cellcept to get me healthy enough again. I continued to eat poorly. I've never been an overweight person, but my body fat must have been 20% or higher. For me that is really high. I was able to return to work but struggled with the threat of another flare up for almost two years. I remained healthy enough to maintain my medical and work safely, but not enough to challenge myself.

Then on November 15th 2002, I met Colin Abrams. My wife and I were taking her grandparents to Orlando, Florida as they were unable to drive this year due to advancing age. They bought three tickets on the airline I work for and I had booked the jump seat. The jump seat is a "spare" seat in the flight deck reserved for check airman and FAA personnel to conduct line checks and observations. If the seat is unoccupied, qualified company flight deck personnel (pilots) may occupy it. We were on a Boeing 727, a three pilot aircraft. The second officer (flight engineer) was a bright, enthusiastic pilot named Colin. His duties are much lighter during cruise flight and we struck up a conversation. As it turns out he has a PhD in natural medicine. We started talking about arthritis and causes and effects. I was curious what he would say about a disease in the same family as mine. He spoke very intelligently and I soon told him of my illness and frustrations with it. He proceeded to give me a free seminar on cell function, disease, causes and corrections. I had notes on the backs of envelopes and weather briefings. He advised me on good ways to get started towards a healthier lifestyle and then a healthier life.

My wife and I started the moment we deplaned in Orlando. In a few short months I have gone from struggling to complete 1000 yard swims to powering through 3500 yard swims and holding myself back for fear of too much, too fast. I also lift light weights with high reps for muscular balance. My body fat has dropped from 18% to 13% and continues to do so while my calories increase. My metabolism seems to be at a level I have not seen since prior to 1996. I sleep better, think better, look better and have the confidence to know the disease I have or side effects of the meds I take, will no longer prevent me from seeing the child my wife is carrying in her womb be born, go to school, graduate, marry, struggle and succeed in life. As I look back at the biggest accomplishment of my life, swimming the Straights of Mackinaw, I realize I was eating similar to what I eat now. I was doing it because I was in a training mentality. Now, I am in a healthy body mentality and I am enthused about every meal because I know it is one step closer to good health. Somewhere along the line my immune system did not like something in my environment. It could have been any number of things. A pet, my diet, my apartment, my on-demand charter flying with all night (and day) schedules, a flu virus or any number of things. I have a history of an abnormal immune system with allergies as a young child. Now, I am giving my body what it needs to function properly as well as staying away from the things that may make it run astray.

What follows is a typical day in my life of eating right and supplementing. I will try to explain as best I can with my limited knowledge of cell function and interactions. Colin told me I could find these supplements at most health food stores. We all seem to want a doctor to give us a pill to make us better, but we don't always use the discipline to take care of ourselves. I can tell you it is much easier to lead a disciplined, healthy lifestyle than to be sick and tired all the time. I stop by the market twice a week for about 15 minutes each time. Cooking is simple. Everything tastes fresh and great. Clean up is easy and I am amazed at how much cupboard space we now have that all of our refined foods are gone. Every meal is a treat that will power me to my next workout or a great night of sleep. I can't over state my enthusiasm for this and I hope your results are as good as mine.

If we need a snack we will have fruit, carrots, cheese (aged over 90 days), sprouted grain bread or my favourite .... home-made trail mix. I put in a mix of raisins and almonds (for favourable pH balance) with cashews, walnuts, soy nuts, filberts, peanuts etc. We do not drink tap water. It has additives and chemicals I do not want in my body. We drink only pure, filtered water and drink lots of it. We usually add a bit of lemon or lime to help keep our bodies pH balanced. We do not drink dairy as our bodies are not designed to digest milk after a young age. We get our calcium from the foods we eat and supplement with coral calcium. We do not eat refined foods such as flours, sugars etc. For the most part we only eat fresh, whole foods. Coffee is now a treat to me. I may allow myself a cup once or twice a week, but no more. Decaf is not an option as the process they use adds harsh chemicals I do not want in my body. We do not eat or drink anything that has artificial sweeteners.

I supplement as follows:

A probiotic helps to detox the digestive tract. The refined foods we eat (flours, sugars etc.) clog our system up and can cause a variety of health problems.

A systemic enzyme – your body produces systemic enzymes. However, as we age we lose some of our ability to produce the amount we need. The enzyme makes up the difference and better allows us to heal and function normally (as people with inflammatory diseases, our immune systems do not function normally).

Calcium – calcium is the most common mineral in our body. It aids in many processes and helps to maintain proper pH balance. Coral calcium is the best form of it. Lots of easily assimilated calcium with trace minerals.

Flaxseed oil – we need omega 3's and 6's to build good cells. Without them we build weaker cells that may dysfunction. This is a great way to be certain we are getting what we need.

Multi-vitamin and mineral – a nutrient dense supplement to be certain we are getting the things we need if we do not get it from our diet.

That is what is working for me and it is working wonders. Please go to Colin's website *www.bodiesbydocmurdoc.com* and poke around a bit. Read his articles, they are enlightening. As I said, Colin is bright,enthused, sincere and knowledgeable. He's a former Olympian (short track cycling), a major airline pilot and a good guy. You can contact him through his website. I highly recommend the services of someone like him as it has changed my life. My physicians never once mentioned my diet or ways to help myself through nutrition. All I was told was 3 square meals a day.

My diet and supplements are also a work in progress as I mix and match to try to fine tune things a bit for me. If you think it is difficult to make this complete, dedicated change to your lifestyle, think about how hard it was to lift your head off the pillow this morning or wash your hair, play with your child, get out of the car. I know how hard it is to do those things with DM. I nearly lost my career and means of supporting myself to this disease. Many of you have lost more than that. Instead, I found a partner in dermatomyositis to challenge me and keep me interested and fascinated with life. That brings me to my last point. I REFUSE TO BE A VICTIM OF THIS ILLNESS (OR ANY OTHER!). I may be sick, but I don't have to let it win. My immune system will probably always have the ability to attack me. I'm fine with that. I have no other choice. If I sit on the couch and feel sorry for myself (and I have at times) I will not get better. Some days, that was the most energy I had. However, I could eat right and start a journey toward achievement. When I enter that triathlon this spring, it is not to beat the person next to me. I will likely never have that ability again. I enter to beat the idea that I shouldn't enter. I want to beat the idea that my doctor thought I should take long walks and possibly give up aviation. I want to beat the concept that someone with my disease can't do triathlons. I want to beat the fact that I was training for a triathlon 7 years ago when I first became sick. I want to beat that little bit of self-doubt that says I may not be able to finish. I do not care where I place among my 'peers'. It may take me all day, but I will finish. That is how God designed me. It is how my parents raised me. It is what life has taught me. Lastly, I do not want to look at my child someday from a wheel chair. This is perhaps the greatest motivator I have ever known. The most important task in my life (fatherhood) is finally upon me and I do not have the luxury of failing. I challenge you as I challenge myself to 'Never Give Up!'

A word about exercise – the level of physical exercise I seek is not a good idea for all people with DM. Before I was sick, I was a fit person. Therefore, I had a foundation of physical fitness. My first 'workout' toward health and the Straights of Mackinaw was a walk of about 100 yards with my older brother. A few days later, I went maybe 110 yards. My current fitness level was built over a period of a couple of years. If a person with myositis were to start into an exercise regimen too quickly, the results would likely be disastrous. We must start slowly and work our way up. We must pay attention to our body and what it is communicating. If I felt 'off' or not up to my training on a particular day, I would adjust its intensity or duration or perhaps I would just wait another day. I never hesitated to program in another day of rest if I needed one. I have tried to challenge my illness, yet not anger it. In this way, DM and I have worked together to make the gains we have. Take your time and build gradually. Learn how your body responds. Take the time to discover what type of exercise and at what level will work for you.

My best wishes to you all and of course - ' Never Give Up!'

Update June 2005

This is an update to the letter I wrote my for fellow myositis patients in early 2003. Since that time, my life has changed dramatically. Most significantly, our son was born and is rapidly approaching his second birthday. We are also blessed to be pregnant with our second child. My health continues to be a non-issue in our lives. I was able to taper off all meds on April 1, 2003. We have continued our healthy lifestyle and I have been able to compete in bike races, triathlons and most importantly, play with my energetic little boy. In late July of 2004, I swam the Straights of Mackinaw again. This time, I was med free. In many ways it was a greater achievement than the first time in 1999. I was on prednisone and methotrexate then. Now, I remain med free and asymptomatic. Dermatomyositis is no longer a limiting factor in my life or the life of my family. It is still with us as a motivator, an achievement and a reminder of how precious the gift of good health is to my family.

Our diet has been slightly refined from my previous writing, but largely the same. I still confer with Dr. Colin Abrams (now an MD as well as PhD) on a regular basis. I continue my exercise regimen with my emphasis on endurance training. My favourite activity is road cycling with a routine of light resistance, high repetition weights for my upper body fitness. My attitude remains the same. I am not, nor will I ever be a victim of this disease (or any other). Oddly enough, I am thankful for its inclusion in my life. Everything I do or see is more precious now. My wife and son, our unborn child, a 40 mile bike ride, downhill skiing with my parents, or a beautiful sunrise, all have a deeper significance than I previously imagined. I am grateful to my wife and children, my parents and God for all they do to teach, motivate, lead, and inspire.

I hope this small glimpse into my struggle with DM over the last nine and a half years is helpful to you in your challenge. Keep a positive attitude and 'Never Give Up!'

Rae   PM
70 years old. Diagnosed aged 67.

In 2002 I was diagnosed with polymyositis after months of muscle weakness and fatigue that I didn't understand. When my neuro-doc said the only treatment for this incurable disease was long-term use of prednisone, I was alarmed.

He also said that after age 60, (I was 66) it MAY stop the inflammation but it could take a year to find out!

Seven years ago, my husband, a pediatrician now retired, and I went into a home-based business that deals with alternative health products for prevention of disease and for improving the quality of life of people who already have problems. Up to that time, we had never believed in anything unscientific. My husband has had a huge paradigm shift in his thinking, as have I, realizing that Eastern medicine understands the body better than Western. We treat symptoms; they treat the CAUSE. We have met so many people who have been cured or just helped with all kinds of alternative therapies that we decided it was a worth a try to find an alternative treatment for polymyositis.

When I told the doctor that that was the route I wanted to take, he said, "I can't direct you because I don't know anything about alternatives, but I do know what steroids do to you and I don't blame you. Come back in two months and I will monitor you." I was thrilled.

I have done a number of things and you must understand that it is all out-of-pocket expenses. What I think has worked and is working is going to a Naturopath (since September 2002) who finds all kinds of things that are wrong inside and gives remedies to fix them. She calls it "peeling the layers of an onion", and every month or so she finds that one thing is healed and something else shows up. Very interesting. She also does darkfield microscopy, which looks at your blood and can diagnose other problems. Fascinating. Watching my blood become healthy over several months was awesome!

The other major thing is amino acid therapy from The Canadian Cancer Research Group (CCRG) in Canada. You send them your blood plasma and they study it in lots of ways, particularly for your amino acids. Then they make up a compound DESIGNED FOR YOU to correct the highs and lows. I expected this all to take only about 6 months to work, but in 6 months I was only a little less fatigued. But, when I went back to the doc to see what he had to say (wasn't sure if I had gotten weaker or not), he said he thought I had stayed the same for the last 3 months (!) and my CPK had dropped from 3900 to 2410. I was ecstatic, and decided to continue. Oh, I have been pain-free from the beginning.

In March my energy started coming back noticeably, and now, April 2004, it's back big time. Also the CCRG had promised that my muscles would repair and they are doing just that! In addition, I am using a homeopathic remedy to detox mercury and heavy metals from my body. In May 2003 I started seeing a massage therapist twice a week for light massage and after a few months she started stretching my muscles and giving me exercises to do at home. I give her credit for all the physical abilities that I am regaining almost weekly.

On January 6th 2004 my neuro-doc and I agreed that I don't need to see him anymore! He is amazed at how I have recovered. I am still not 100% back to where I was but maybe 85% and still improving.

You can go to *www.ccrg.com* and read about the Canadian group. It only talks about cancer, but they feel that once your body is cleared up of whatever is wrong, you will heal….whatever the disease.

And that's what I'm doing.

Update June 2005

I am doing incredibly well. I feel 'normal' again. I have returned to my exercise class twice a week (and I have to walk up a flight of steps to the class), and there is very little I am unable to do. We all work at our own pace, but I am very pleased with my physical abilities. I'll be 70 in a few weeks! People who didn't see me when I was "sick" have no idea that I ever was.

My CPK has been totally normal since July. As a matter of fact, when I was told in July 2004 that it was 101, I was in disbelief and had it drawn again at another lab. 75!

I don't know if it is remission, or what. (At my age, it could be a cure!) But my husband and I each have our lives back.

Just another interesting piece of information – my neuromuscular doctor told me that muscles don't regenerate after 60 years old. I am proof that he was wrong!

Peter   DM
61 years old. Diagnosed aged 58.

I was diagnosed with dermatomyositis in January 2001 and was treated with prednisolone and methotrexate.
Coping with tapering prednisolone was not difficult as the reduction made me feel better and less hungry. Towards the end I needed to add methotrexate as the prednisolone was not controlling the skin rashes. Coping with tapering methotrexate was not as easy, as the skin rashes came back a little and now I am off the methotrexate I am left with itchy areas. I had to come off the methotrexate as it was affecting my liver, indicated by a high P3NP blood count.
I have been in remission for 12 months with no sign of the muscle weakness returning but I have itchy areas of skin that cannot be scratched as they become very sore.

Update 6 months later

I have less itchy skin now after finding the right cream. The muscle weakness is returning a little. Otherwise things are fine.

Dee   DM
49 years old. Diagnosed aged 40.

"Life begins at 40."
  Whoever said that, wants shooting!
  Exactly five weeks after my 40th birthday, I was diagnosed with dermatomyositis. I was experiencing flu-like symptoms upon my return from a surprise birthday week in Kenya organised by my husband. I actually felt unwell on holiday, but put it down to the heat (the tem-

perature was in the 90's). My GP was on the ball, and listened carefully to my explanation of symptoms and organised some blood tests including CPK; something not many GP's would pick up on. A week later, I visited my GP feeling considerably worse; he told me I was very ill and needed to be hospitalised immediately for further investigations. Five days later the diagnosis was made. I was numb! I couldn't absorb this news. They have made a mistake. I have just got flu. I cried for days and was in denial. I left hospital in a wheelchair, still not realising my prognosis. I came home surrounded by cards and flowers, but was still in a total state of shock and disbelief. It was surreal.

I was started on a regime of 60 mg of prednisolone and azathioprine immediately and within six months I was so fat and bloated, I hardly recognised myself in the mirror. Who was this woman; it wasn't me? People I had known for years didn't recognise me. I felt like a freak and became a recluse. There is so much fear around illness. People see you not as a person, but a disease. Fortunately, I have moved on since then and I can forgive those that were scared to face me.

The greatest loss for me was my job in December 1996. After six months, my employment was terminated, which left me with no self worth or purpose in life. The New Year saw me referred for counselling assessment. I was told I was not clinically depressed but had a reactive depression as a direct result of my illness. I was so relieved. Somehow, I had the strength to make counselling work for me. I had a lot of insight into my situation. This was to be the most significant turning point. We explored a lot of issues and got to a point where I could move forward and start living again. We talked about how I would move forward and pursue an Aromatherapy course. That has been one of the best decisions I have ever made.

Everyone around me wondered how I could even contemplate learning something physical with the fatigue that would be involved. Typically, that's like a red rag to a bull. I'm just like a kid – if someone says don't, I do it! However, this decision proved to be the best I have ever made career-wise. In fact, it helped me to recover physically and my muscles became stronger, not weaker. This was to be just the beginning! I spent the next three years studying other therapies, then I did a two-year teaching certificate and trained to be an Assessor of complementary therapies; my career went from strength to strength.

In June 1998, I had another appointment to see my consultant at Kings College Hospital. This visit was to be the beginning of the rest of my life. By now, hospital appointments were becoming predictable. Over a period of time, the process of gradually weaning me off prednisolone and azathioprine filled me with neither anxiety nor excitement. It just happened. This visit was different. I wasn't expecting to leave his consulting room elated. But I did! He told me almost as soon as I sat down that I no longer needed to take anymore medication as he felt I was in remission. It was complete and utter disbelief. I had never expected to hear that word. I thought steroids etc. were going to continue to be part of my everyday life. He then said he didn't need to see me again for 6 months unless I had any problems.

In August 2001, I started my job as an Aromatherapist to set up a complementary therapy service for people with cancer. The service has grown and developed beyond my expectations, as has my role. I now work two days per week at a Cancer Unit (within an NHS hospital) and I have extended the service to the local hospice. Patients can now access complementary therapies from diagnosis to end stage disease.

My experiences of living with a life-threatening illness have given me the skills and empathy to do the work I am doing today. This may sound trite, but I know I was meant to have dermatomyositis for a reason. Often, patients say to me "you always know exactly what I need, how do you do that?" I guess it's innate within me and I have always worked with my instincts and gut feeling. Having dermatomyositis has taken me to places I had never expected to be during my forties. I see my patients in those same places though often, much younger. I can look back now and actually see DM as being a positive experience, only because I am lucky enough to have been in remission for seven years now. Without this experience, I wouldn't be the person I am today; I wouldn't be doing the job I do and be motivated to push myself to achieve my goals. Most of all, to fight for my health so I could be with my family and see all the things every mother wants to see, like children going to university, getting married, and experiencing the joys of being a grandparent. Nine years ago I didn't know if I would experience any of those things. But, thankfully, I have.

I have a history of rheumatoid arthritis dating back to 1991, which was in remission before I developed DM and now the DM is in remission, the RA is back. I have always had homeopathic treatment for the RA. It keeps it under control without having to resort to cytotoxic medications. This is my main challenge health-wise. I am not sure which is worse, the fatigue through muscle weakness or the excruciating pain of inflamed joints.

One of my main problems with DM was dealing with the distressing, unwanted side- effects of steroids. Body image, self-esteem, confidence had all taken a bashing. Even though I still carry excess weight, I can live with myself; I like myself and most of the time my self-esteem is intact. I can look at myself in the mirror and not be repulsed by what I see. What puts it into perspective for me now is seeing patients who have had invasive, mutilating surgery and treatments for cancer and how their altered body image affects their daily lives and causes so much distress.

I am very aware the outcome for everyone is not so good and I am grateful every day I feel well. I will never have the energy I had before DM, but I have a good quality of life and I am happy with that. Having DM and working with cancer patients makes me realise that life is so short and fragile and certainly, for me, I have to make the most of it. I am determined to live life to the full, because tomorrow it could all go pear-shaped again. I have no regrets as I have done so much since having DM. I don't know if I would have otherwise.

Sometimes, I have to remind myself that I am not cured; I am only in remission and that the disease could rear its ugly head at anytime. Meanwhile, I will continue to live a productive, fulfilling life, helping people to cope and come to terms with life-threatening illness. I have come to terms with many of the issues I faced dealing with DM and I never forget how far I have come. It has been a difficult journey, but with a lot of support from family and friends, I feel I have come out the other side. Remission is a good place to be!

In nine months time I shall be 50; there was a time when I thought I would not see this milestone. My next challenge? Well, instead of opting for a quiet life, true to type, I'm thinking of embarking upon a master's degree course this September. Whether I do it or not, I hope to realise the challenge of attaining my half-century!

Karen   **PM**
61 years old. Diagnosed aged 37.

My story of having polymyositis started back in January 1980. After having a wonderful holiday, I became sick with what was probably flu. I believe, because my resistance was low at that time, the beginning of polymyositis started to emerge.

At first I had difficulties going up and down stairs and then my hands were so stiff in the morning I couldn't even hold a knife or fork. As time went on, I had difficulty getting out of chairs, holding a hair dryer, and some mornings getting out of bed. I eventually went to the doctors.

My doctor, who was a rheumatology specialist, at first thought I had Lupus. After blood tests, a muscle biopsy, and an electromyogram (EMG), I was told I had polymyositis. This was a shock to me as I had never heard of this disease. I was 37 years old and had always been very healthy.

I was immediately put on very high doses of the steroid prednisone. For 8 years I experienced a roller coaster ride taking prednisone and methotrexate. Finally, after a long time of being on a very low dose of prednisone, my doctor decided to try and take me completely off steroids. This worked…and still is working!!

My doctor told me, there is nothing I can do or avoid doing to prevent the onset of coming out of remission. There is no comprehensible explanation or reason given why or how this disease can become active again.

It took a while for my "moon face" to disappear and some of the weight to come off from taking prednisone for such a long time. I'm still reminded at times that I have this disease. If I was to bump my arm or upper leg, it's very painful. Going up stairs is a little difficult for me. My hands are sometimes stiff and I still experience mild effects of Raynaud's disease. At times getting out of chairs can be a little difficult. I do find if I kneel down for any reason, I have to lean on a chair, bed, etc. to help push myself up.

I find myself checking for signs of my disease coming back. I do have a physical every year and my blood level (CPK) is always checked. So far it has remained normal. I remember, whenever my doctor lowered my prednisone dosage I usually knew if I was getting worse before he would get the blood test results.

I do walk a lot, enjoy golfing and know my limitations. My husband retired and we are now living and loving our life in sunny Florida. Sometimes it's hard to look back and remember all that I went through. I was in some ways lucky: my disease was caught early and I never had any permanent muscle damage.

It's been a long time since 1980, a time when this disease was not well known. I really felt alone and having to take prednisone I felt depressed at times.

This book is really a great source of support for many people. It lets us see we are not alone.

Tom DM
49 years old. Diagnosed aged 44.

My name is Tom and I live in southern Massachusetts. I was diagnosed with dermatomyositis in October of 2000.

I first noticed that something was wrong with me in the summer of 2000. I was 44 years old at the time and had kept myself in excellent shape. I would run 20-25 miles a week; sometimes as far as 10 miles at a time. However, in late June of 2000, on one particular day, I went running and noticed that something was wrong. I just didn't feel right. It is hard to describe but I had a hazy unbalanced feeling. I gave up the run and walked home. Later that day I suffered from very tight muscle cramps in my legs. These symptoms seem to be particular to me, because I have not heard of anyone else that first noticed myositis by feeling unbalanced and hazy.

From that day forward I became gradually worse. My running distance got less and less as I slowly got weaker and weaker. By late July I knew there was something not right and I went to my family doctor. My doctor ran a number of blood tests and noticed that my liver enzymes were elevated. He told me to stop drinking alcohol, although I wasn't a heavy drinker to begin with. I went back to him a month later and back again two weeks later. I continued to feel worse and worse. It was like I had a hangover and if I just got enough sleep I would feel better, but no amount of sleep made me feel better. By early fall I was so weak I could not do a modified push up (knees on the ground) and running was out of the question. At one point I was so miserable I confined myself to bed for a few days. I honestly considered the possibility that I was going to die.

During this time I went to see a number of other doctors, including a doctor of internal medicine and a neuro-musculoskeletal doctor. None of them could make a diagnosis. Finally, on the last day of October 2000, I went to see a rheumatologist. He diagnosed me in about 30 seconds. He was familiar with myositis and recognized the symptoms. One of the things I thought odd was that he looked in my eyes and said, "Yes, I think you have myositis". I said, "The only part of me still working is my eyes. What makes you see myositis in my eye?" He said, "Myositis affects all your muscles and the muscle in your eye will show a purple ring when it is inflamed."

I had a blood test the next day and a muscle biopsy two days later. My blood test showed I had a CPK of 2700. The muscle biopsy gave the definitive result of dermatomyositis. My doctor put me on 60 mg of prednisone a day. I also went on disability. After being on prednisone for 4 weeks, my CPK was still 1500, so the rheumatologist put me on 20 mg/week of methotrexate.

Prednisone has to be one of the nastiest drugs available. Up until my diagnosis, I was pretty much bed ridden. Once I went on prednisone, I did not sleep for the first 48 hours. After that, for the next two weeks, I slept about 3 hours a night. Then my body adjusted to the prednisone and I crashed. I slept for the next week.

I kept a daily log from the time I was diagnosed until today. I tracked my medication, my exercise and how I felt on a day to day basis. The first few months of this disease after diagnosis were very difficult. I don't know if it was the disease or the prednisone, or both, but it was the most difficult time of my life. I ultimately lost about 25 pounds from my running weight. I also had periods of misery, where I spent days in bed. I gradually got adjusted and went back to work part time in early 2001, but 2001 was still the worst year of my life. I wrote in my log in early 2001 that getting up in the morning, I would have no idea how my day would go. There were days that I would get in the car to drive to work and turn around and go home, feeling so bad that I should not be driving a car.

Throughout 2001, my doctor and I tried to reduce my dose of prednisone. By the end of July 2001, I was able to come off of prednisone completely and was only on methotrexate.

Over the next two and a half years we continued to work to reduce the methotrexate. I would reduce my dosage by 2.5 mg every time I had three consecutive months of a CPK below 200. Twice I had a flare in which I had to have my dosage of methotrexate increased, one time almost back to my original dose. However, over time this disease seemed to burn itself out. By December of 2003 I managed to come off of all drugs and I have been drug free ever since.

Throughout my ordeal with dermatomyositis I worked to try to get my body back in shape. Once diagnosed and on medication, my weight was down to 149 pounds (from 175). My strength was terrible and my endurance was worse. Once my CPK was continually below 200 (starting around March of 2001), I went to physical therapy and then started taking beginners yoga classes. It was a long slow process to get my body back in shape. I am still working on this today.

Like I said, I came off all drugs in December of 2003 and have managed to stay off all medication to this day. I am not where I was five years ago, but I continue to work to get my mind and body back in shape. I have had periods of time when I was sure the myositis was back because I was feeling so poorly, but all tests have come up negative and eventually the feeling went away. For the most part I am feeling pretty good. I can run 3 miles and I do power yoga a couple times a week.

Chronic illness not only affects your body, but your mind as well. Being unhealthy for a long period of time can be as much a mental battle as a physical one. It is hard to lose your health for a long period of time and not become depressed. It is hard not to feel all alone when you are chronically ill.

I continue to work hard at yoga and running and appreciate every day that I have. People around me have no idea that I was ever sick. I have gone to a number of mental health doctors to fight depression. The reason why I have seen a number of them is because most mental health doctors do not understand the burden of chronic illness.

Today I have to say that I am a very lucky man. I am healthy and active. My son is going to college this fall. I have managed to maintain my career throughout this ordeal and for the most part I feel excellent.

Good luck to all of you out there fighting myositis.

Diane   DM
32 years old. Diagnosed aged 23.

I've been in remission for 8 years now after what I'd consider a severe flare.

I was diagnosed in October 1996 at the age of 23.

It began with a horrible pain in my calves plus an itchy rash on my thighs. Within one week I would nearly pass out if I attempted to move from my bedroom to the couch. It progressed to involve difficulties swallowing, breathing and just about every muscle in my body was affected. I choked down nothing but baby food for two months. I could not lift my head off a pillow nor muster the energy to shower myself. Watching TV was even too hard for me to do.

I was put on high dose prednisone daily – and then methotrexate was added after the first few months. My prednisone taper took a little over a year and the methotrexate went a few months beyond that. I was so scared every time I lowered the dosage because my muscle pain would crop up for the first few days...but by the 4th day it felt like such a victory! I was able to go back to work part-time after exactly 6 months, full time 2 months after that.

I have been in a medication free remission for say seven years now. My life has been completely normal. My muscle strength never made it back to where it was pre-DM, like I struggle to do squats but it hasn't slowed me down much...I've done cardio-kickboxing, got certified for SCUBA and ridden horses...

Update July 2005

I'm doing great and leading a normal life. Honestly, I rarely even think of the disease that turned my life upside down nearly a decade ago.

Jenny   DM
55 years old. Diagnosed aged 47.

It's been a rocky road but I made it.

When I was diagnosed in June 1998 my consultant told me that it would be a minimum of two years on steroids. In June 2000 he told me that I was well enough to stop taking them. I was in remission. Funnily enough it was a lovely sunny day just like the day I had been diagnosed. I was ecstatic. I drove home with music playing full blast; singing my head off. What I didn't know was that it was going to be another four years before I got off steroids.

My adrenal glands had decided to go to sleep. Below 10mg of prednisolone, whenever I tried reducing just 1mg, I nearly collapsed with exhaustion. I had an ACTH / Synacthen Test to check my adrenal function and the endocrinologist said the result showed that I would probably have to stay on a low dose of steroids for the rest of my life. I was no longer ecstatic. I felt awful most days and struggled to work part-time.

I must say at this point that the majority of people do not experience major problems tapering steroids. As long as you taper slowly, as your consultant will advise, then you should be fine. I was just unlucky.

Anyway, I worked out a regime of tapering the steroids that I could cope with. I tapered just 1 mg over 8 weeks, sometimes going back up to my original dose if I felt unwell.

I would stay on the tapered dose for a couple of months before repeating the process again. I continued like this until I got to 5mg. However, when I tried to go from 5mg to 4mg, I couldn't do it, the withdrawal symptoms were awful. I was then changed to hydrocortisone. Hydrocortisone has a shorter half life than prednisolone (stays in your blood for less time) and mimics your natural corticosteroid rhythm more accurately. I started on 20mg of hydrocortisone (20mg of hydrocortisone is equivalent to 5mg of prednisolone in effect). I took it twice a day (10mg/dose at 7am and 3pm). This helped to kick start my adrenal response. I also spent a day in hospital where they measured my natural cortisol levels every hour. I tapered the hydrocortisone over 5 months, eventually coming off steroids in February 2004.

Since then the DM has stayed in remission. All my blood tests are normal.

Mentally I found dealing with DM difficult. I think it is almost like a bereavement. When you eventually get a diagnosis you feel optimistic that you have a name for your condition and that it is not 'all in your head'. You are going to be taken seriously. Then the reality sinks in. Your life changes radically. You have to deal with your looks changing as well coming to terms mentally with having a chronic illness.

My own experience was to gain two stone in weight, look like a chipmunk, watch my skin and hair become thin and basically not like what I saw in the mirror. I did suffer depression to some extent, two years into the illness, and this was exacerbated when my mother died in 2003. I definitely didn't want anti-depressants and so I went to a counsellor for two years. I found this to be an enormous help and would recommend others who find depression getting on top of them to follow this route. On the bright side, I have now lost all the weight with the help of Weight Watchers, my hair is becoming thick again and I can see the 'old me' when I look in the mirror!

Last year I cycled in Norfolk and did thirty five miles! Admittedly I was lost, but was amazed that I could do it. My strength is back to normal and I can walk up hill and down without experiencing any muscle weakness. I am thrilled to have been drug-free for over two years and view my DM as a thing of the past. I hope it helps people who have recently been diagnosed with myositis, to read these positive stories on remission.

The worst thing about having DM
Fatigue

The best thing about having DM
My wonderful 'new' friends.

What are my tips to reach remission?
- Listen to your consultant.
- Discuss your treatment and be honest with each other.
- Ask questions if you don't understand your disease/treatment.
- If you are on steroids, taper them VERY slowly and only when told to by your consultant.
- Listen to your body.
- Rest when your body tells you to.
- Exercise as much as you can but don't push yourself. A gentle walk, swimming or cycle ride is plenty. If you are unsure then see a physiotherapist.
- Eat fresh fruit/vegetables daily.

- Eat enough protein.
- See a nutritionist to get dietary advice especially on supplements.
- Join a support group.
- Try to keep your mind active.
- Make goals and have a purpose to your life.
- Find a creative hobby.
- Have someone you can talk to with whom you feel understood and safe.
- Be positive (hard at times, but persevere!)

SECTION TWO

Living with Myositis

5

Is this Myositis?

by Jenny Fenton

One of my main observations of people with myositis is that they are all very different in the symptoms they display. No two of us are alike. Overlap with other autoimmune conditions is common too; thus confusing the origin of the symptom.

After researching this rather 'grey' area I have compiled the following list. Some of the symptoms you will recognise, others you will not. All of these complaints have been reported by a significant number of people with myositis. Whether they are related to the myositis, drug side effects or another condition is up to you to decide with the help of your doctor.

I must emphasize that just because you have myositis it doesn't mean you're going to experience all of these symptoms.

Back pain

Bitter/metallic taste in the mouth

Buffalo hump

Burning sensation in the muscles

Constipation

Cracks and soreness on the cuticles

Depression

Diarrhoea

Difficulty swallowing

Difficulty walking upstairs

Difficulty rising from a chair

Difficulty walking

Dizziness

Double incontinence and urgency

Dry mouth

Excessive thirst

Exhaustion

Facial hair growth

Falling over – losing balance

Hair going completely straight

Hair loss

Heartburn

Heel/Foot pain when getting out of bed

High blood pressure

Indigestion

Lack of sex drive

Loss of body hair

Loss of use of some muscles

Memory loss

Mood swings

Moon face

Muscle pain

Muscle wasting

Muscle weakness

Neck pain

Osteoporosis/Bone loss

Pain at the bottom of the feet

Pain in the shins when walking

Palpitations

Panic attacks

Prickling/Tingling sensations

Puffiness between knuckles

Puffiness on fingers

Rash

Shoulder pain

Skin thinning

Sleeplessness

Sweats

Swollen ankles

Swollen wrists

Throbbing in the thighs

Trembling

Visual disturbances

Weight gain

Weight loss

THE THINGS WE DON'T TALK ABOUT

Depression

Depression seems to go hand in hand with having a chronic illness and I think this is totally justified. From being active, healthy, positive people our lives are suddenly turned upside down and will probably never be quite the same again. On waking in the morning you probably have a second or two before you remember your illness. I personally hate that moment when I realize that things are not what they used to be. Wouldn't it be lovely to wake up and 'just be normal'?

The symptoms of depression can include lack of motivation, waking early and not being able to get to sleep again, avoiding people, excessive sleepiness, lack of self-confidence, changes in appetite and loss of libido.

If depression becomes a major problem you must seek help. There are people out there trained to help (see chapter on counselling). It is not showing a weakness at all – far from it – as I said before it is quite understandable that we will get depressed – who wouldn't?

Counselling can be sought either through your doctor or possibly through a church or other faith institution. Counselling services are often attached to churches and do not cost too much. Often a donation of what you can afford is fine. You don't have to be a church member or belong to any particular faith. Many offer help from anything up to a few weeks to a year. I would recommend going for weekly sessions until you really feel more able to cope – this could take months. The hour per week is for you to laugh, cry or just talk – no one is going to judge you – they will just be there for you. It is your time.

Crying can be a huge release and counselling offers a safe haven to do this privately. Talking is vital when you feel depressed, so that you can express your fear and innermost pain.

Eventually you start to accept your condition, but do other people? It is hard convincing family and friends that on some days, without warning, you will have to pull out of whatever you had arranged. The unpredictability can be very hard on you and our carers and friends. It's often said that having a chronic illness makes you realise who your real friends really are.

Depression can be helped so don't suffer in silence – Talk to someone.

Rectal incontinence

Whether or not this is connected with myositis, drug side effects or neither is debatable.

All I can say is that I have met a significant number of people with myositis for whom this is a problem.

If you do suffer from rectal incontinence then you must talk to your doctor about it so that other conditions can be eliminated. I was found to have coeliac disease. I had suffered all my life with stomach problems and so in some ways it was a relief to find out what had caused them.

Thinking logically I would have thought it is feasible that rectal muscles could be affected as well as the muscles in the arms/legs etc. but (to my knowledge) this has never been documented.

If you do suffer from this problem and no other medical condition is apparent, then I suggest you take the following advice. Always carry around a spare set of underwear with you and always take the opportunity to use the loo when you go out shopping etc. Ask your doctor for advice on diet (maybe see a dietician) and preventative medicine for the times when you are going out for long periods of time and a loo is not going to be readily available. It is an embarrassing problem and something which we would possibly not wish to share with our family. A doctor will help so pluck up courage and go to see them. Remember you won't be the first person they've seen with this problem and certainly not the last.

Loss of libido

Hey folks we're ill! Ask your partner if he/she feels like sex when they've got flu? Gosh this is a difficult one. How can we 'feel in the mood' when we feel under the weather from time to time? I suppose just grab the moment when you feel well. I expect the chemicals that are released might just even make us feel a little better! You need a very understanding partner to help with this one, as it is certainly not easy. Relationship problems can occur as a result. This is another area that can be helped with counselling (possibly for both of you).

Apparently up to 40% of women and 30% of men experience a loss of libido at some time in their lives so we're not the only ones with this problem. A good sex life is fantastic when both partners are fit and healthy but during the times when our libido is less than adequate, keep the romance going with kind words to each other and affection. A big hug can keep me going for days and makes me feel a million dollars. It's so important to feel loved even if you don't have regular sex – and at the end of the day who does? I think they're all lying.

If all else fails, why not have a romantic, relaxing weekend away which can be a great way to get to know each other again, try to forget about the illness and indulge yourselves. That's my excuse anyway!

Loss of hair (body and head)

I don't think we all experience this but some of us do and it needs to be addressed. It seems to be exacerbated by the illness and some of the drugs we have to take. For a woman it may be nice not to need to shave your legs or under your arms any more but it can be rather disconcerting losing your pubic hair. For a man it can be equally upsetting as hair can be a sign of masculinity. I guess we just need to put things in perspective – worse things happen to some unfortunate people and most of it is only noticeable to us or our partners whom I hope are understanding.

Losing or having thinning hair on your head is also hard to come to terms with. Both women and men who once had lovely thick hair can find their hair goes listless and thin. Women often have to have it cut short. Find a good hairdresser who has had experience with this problem. For women it might be fun to have some colour put in and it can make you feel more 'alive'.

Panic attacks

Why some of us get these I don't know, but lots of us do. It could be a fear of suddenly feeling ill in a public place and not knowing how we will cope. It could also be a culmination of many sleepless nights or acute anxiety about your condition. The symptoms can come on quickly without warning and are extremely frightening. You may experience nausea, palpitations, sweating, the shakes, confusion and a sense of impending doom. You will probably feel embarrassed and try to hide the symptoms. Try to avoid situations where you are more likely to experience an attack. It could be in a hot, crowded room or on a bus, tube or in a train.

Learn some relaxation techniques and breathing exercises. Yoga, Pilates, The Alexander Technique and T'ai Chi are all proven to help.

If you find yourself hyperventilating (over-breathing) then discretely breath into your cupped hands for only a few minutes or better still a paper bag (if available).

The 'Bach Flower Rescue Remedy' is good for helping with panic attacks if used as soon as you feel an attack coming on.

Bleeding Gums

Since I started steroids I have suffered from many gum infections which have had to be treated with local antibiotics. My dentist says they are caused by my weakened immune system. I see the dental hygienist regularly to try to keep my gums in tiptop condition. She gave me a tip which I have found very helpful. I immerse my two toothbrushes in a Milton (used for sterilising babies' bottles) solution every night, which kills off the bacteria that may be harbouring on my toothbrushes. Since doing this my gums have improved enormously. The 'Milton' solution should be changed every three or four days.

See 'Useful Resources' at the back of the book for further help.

6

Emotions, Empathy and Encouragement

Compiled by Jenny Fenton

I f you are reading this it is likely that you have been diagnosed with myositis or that someone close to you has been, or you have a professional interest. To be told that you have a chronic illness brings with it many different emotions. You may be experiencing denial, 'why me?', anger or self-pity, but hopefully eventually you will come to terms with having a chronic illness and find the strength to cope. During my illness I have experienced all these emotions and more. I have turned to various people for help including family and friends but most of all I have talked to other people with myositis. They are the ones who have probably helped and encouraged me the most as they know what it is like. The following are comments made by people with myositis. Some are full of despair, others give you hope. Whatever stage you are at with your myositis you will be able to identify with some of the comments below. If you are feeling despondent try to read and gain strength from the more positive messages – it does help.

I still cling to the hope that it will go away.

What the heck do I have to do to get people to understand the length of fatigue, pain, lack of endurance etc?

I feel like a plant that needs watering.

I think I will live to be a hundred!

'You look fine.' This is the hardest thing to hear.

I am scared about this thing I know nothing about.

It ain't as bad as you think!

Will I see my children grow up? If I can get them to university then they will be OK.

I know I have a mild case but gosh it still hurts!

I want to tell everyone starting out with myositis that it often seems hopeless but don't give up, there is a lot of help out there.

The disease is nasty but the cure is equally bad.

The tiredness for me was 90% withdrawal from prednisolone.

My biggest help was remaining positive – you CAN beat the disease.

This disease can control your mind at times and I hate it.

I want to be free from its power.

I was always very shy and lacked confidence but this disease has forced me to fight with all my might and I have come out of it a much stronger person.

Does anyone ever just cry because they wish they could be normal sometimes?

I am feeling overwhelmed.

It has been a hard six months but I am now climbing stairs and even driving short distances.

It is so hard to accept help and ask for help.

I guess I need a pep talk from someone who has been through this.

The message is that a diagnosis of myositis is not necessarily a life sentence.

I have been so depressed lately that all I want to do is sleep.

I just feel that no one really understands how I feel.

I was elated that I finally had an answer.

People around me have such perfect lives.

I feel so all alone.

I just wanted to say how much better I am feeling. A couple of months ago I was so afraid I thought I was dying. I really understand how hard it is to deal with this and try to live a 'normal' life. But if I can do it – anyone can!

I try very hard not to cry too often. I try to restrain my tears, pretend to sleep, keep myself to myself and hide my feelings.

I'm having a hard time convincing my family/friends that this is a REAL disease.

I feel almost 'normal'. Last year I was looking at motorised scooters and stair-lifts, now you would not know anything was wrong!

It is so hard to deal with this problem and live a 'normal' life.

I want so much to be like I once was.

Some people might think I'm crazy but I'm thrilled to know what I have and feel very hopeful after meeting with all the doctors.

It is hard to accept that I may never be like I used to be.

My whole body seems to droop.

'Attitude' is a major consideration in overcoming myositis.

Is there anything out there that would help with this fatigue?

I am really afraid because I feel like I can't go on the way I am right now and I need some help.

If it wasn't for the inconvenience and frustration of this damn thing it could almost be considered an honour to be a member of such a small, elitist group.

I just want to laugh again.

I'm surprised at how miserable one can feel even when your CK is normal.

Basically I was told that it is all in my head.

I did the shopping today for the first time in months (all by myself!)

Sometimes I feel I'm all washed up and I'm only 30!

I have accepted it as a permanent part of my life.

I thought I could handle almost anything but I never considered this.

The wonderful friends I have made make up for having this lousy disease.

I am taking one day at a time.

Raising my steroids makes me crazy, lowering it wipes me out; I feel like I'm on a constant emotional roller coaster.

I was diagnosed fifteen years ago and am still going strong!

I am sick of hurting all of the time, I am sick of being chubby, I am sick of it all.

What a roller coaster ride this has been; I tell you I'm about ready to get off this train!

Looking back I can't believe that five years ago I couldn't even comb my hair. Talking on the telephone exhausted me, as did climbing the stairs. Now I can walk for miles, swim lengths and feel and look like a new woman.

'The Arrogance of the Healthy' Dr Robert Buckman

Dr Robert Buckman was diagnosed with dermatomyositis when he was 39 years old. In a recent interview with Theresa Curry in The Outlook (the newsletter of The Myositis Association of America) he talks about 'the arrogance of the healthy'. When recently asked what didn't help him when first diagnosed, he replied, 'Well, what really didn't help is when people sent me magnets or herbal preparations or astrology books. It was appalling. Other demoralizing contributions were recommendations to do this or that or theories on what I should have done before to prevent my disease. I call this the arrogance of the healthy. It is the unspoken belief by those who have never suffered from a chronic disease that the disease is somehow the patient's fault. This is natural because people don't want to believe that illness can randomly come to them, that somehow they can prevent it. But it is damaging to the patient.'

Dr Buckman talks about dermatomyositis in his autobiography *'Not Dead Yet'* available through *bookfinder.com* or *amazon.com*.

'Attention to health is life's greatest hindrance.' Plato

A positive attitude may not solve all your problems, but it will annoy enough people to make it worth the effort.' Herm Albright

7

Coping
– stress, relationships and holidays

by Angela Hunter, LMSW,
Myositis Support Group Coordinator, USA

Adapted from open discussions by members of the
Myositis Support Group of the Hospital for Special
Surgery USA December 2004

Coping with Stress When Living with Myositis

Everyone experiences stress, but for those living with rheumatic conditions like myositis, the symptoms of their illness often add an extra layer of complexity to it. For this reason, it may be helpful for those with myositis to enhance or develop coping skills in order to ease the impact of stress on their everyday lives.

The following issues and solutions are summarized from an in–depth and frank discussion by our support group members.

- Medical Appointments
- Social Gatherings
- Riding Public Transportation
- Taking Medications

Medical Appointments

Managing a condition like myositis often requires attending an endless number of doctor appointments by a number of different medical providers. Group members discussed going for physical therapy and IVIG treatments and visiting their rheumatologist, dermatologist, and/or neurologist. These appointments are often scheduled on a regular basis, so you may be going to an appointment related to your myositis every week, or even several times each week. One group member pointed out that appointments related to myositis are in addition to any other regular appointments you should have to monitor your health, such as a mammogram, skin check, or gynaecological examination.

Not only are there many appointments filling up a person's schedule, it can be stressful to figure out transportation to these appointments. This is especially true when you need to be accompanied when travelling, since the schedules of two people need to be consulted. Another way appointments can be stressful is when the doctor is terribly busy with appointments and you have to wait longer than expected. If you have other plans during the day, it can be frustrating to be delayed because an appointment ran late.

Coordinating medical appointments is additionally frustrating when one is experiencing fatigue, a common symptom related to myositis. On the day of an appointment, just getting out of bed and preparing for the day is more complicated when you are fatigued. Also, when it takes longer to get ready for the day, you might find yourself running late. The worry of missing an appointment, the guilt associated with making the doctor wait, or the frustration with oneself for not planning more time can cause great stress and anxiety.

Depending on the nature of the doctor visit, it can be stressful to wait for the doctor to share important news. If you are waiting for the results of a test or if a doctor is considering a new treatment approach, you may be anxious about what you will learn and what it means for you. If you have tried numerous medications, it can be frustrating to see the doctor time after time and learn that a treatment isn't working. Or, if you are experiencing side effects from a medication, it could be upsetting if the doctor insists that you come in right away.

If an appointment is going to result in learning your CPK count, you may feel anxious, since many people with myositis focus on their CPK count as a way to measure any improvement or regression in their health. Patients often worry if their CPK is higher than the previous month's reading or feel relief when they hear it has decreased. As the CPK count rises, group members reported a rise in anxiety, as they fear that it might be an indication that a flare is coming. Even though many people say that it's better to concentrate on how you're feeling and not on the number, it's hard to ignore it when the doctor says it has changed. One group member shared how her number was always fluctuating and she didn't even remember what the normal range was anymore.

Suggestions: One group member said that she always scheduled her doctor's appointment as the first one of the day so that the doctor wasn't busy.

To ease the anxiety of monitoring one's CPK count, one group member suggested writing down the CPK level in a journal and then recording how you are feeling next to it. It will help you track whether or not the level is a good indication of feelings like fatigue or pain. Another group member told the group to ask their doctor to write the CPK level into the file and to discuss it with them only when necessary. If you need to know what your CPK level is, then try not to obsess about the number. Instead, you might want to consult with your medical doctor on ways to lower it.

Social Gatherings

The impact of myositis can complicate one's ability to participate in social gatherings for special occasions, holidays, or work events. For instance, using a wheelchair or a stick/cane to move around can render a person immobile at a crowded party. Not only is it difficult to manoeuver through the crowd, it can be difficult to participate in discussions with other guests when you are stuck in a corner or if everyone else is standing above your wheelchair.

Another difficulty of social gatherings is that they are often held in unfamiliar locations. When friends and family invite you to dinner, to a graduation party, or to a wedding, it can cause you to begin thinking of many concerns related to the accessibility of the location and of the bathroom. People using assistive devices such as a wheelchair or a stick/cane need to be sure that they can manoeuver around. They also need to find out if there is a working lift/elevator if there are too many steps. Some individuals make the decision to decline the invitation rather than deal with the stress of figuring out whether or not they can comfortably attend the gathering.

Entertaining others in one's home takes a lot of time and energy, and several group members shared feelings of regret that they are no longer able to host parties or family gatherings. One group member said she always enjoyed cooking for others by hosting a dinner party. Now, she doesn't have the energy to get the house ready, prepare the food, and then clean up afterwards. Taking the rubbish/garbage out is also a tough chore for someone experiencing muscle weakness. The group discussed their feelings of guilt and disappointment to always be on the receiving end of invitations.

Suggestions: The group discussed how they have to make a greater effort to participate in social gatherings. They may schedule naps on the day of the party or spend extra time resting the day before the gathering. They also prepare themselves for feeling 'wiped out' the day following a social outing and try not to schedule any activities.

For those who really want to invite others to their home but do not have the energy to entertain, a pot-luck lunch could be a fun way to socialize. Also, using paper plates and plastic utensils doesn't require doing the dishes. Most guests are willing to help out, and they would be happy to help take out the rubbish/garbage or help with some light cleaning before leaving. Dinner parties may not be the same as they were before you had myositis, but they can still be fun.

Riding Public Transportation

The buses and underground/subways often seem so convenient, but when muscles are fatigued and you have limitations to your mobility, these transportation options are not always friendly. The group said that the underground/subways always mean lots of stairs. One group member said that she always feels bad for holding up the line at the stairs because it takes her longer to climb them. Another group member often lets buses go by if all the seats up front are taken. After letting two buses pass, the member often decides to walk instead. It can be uncomfortable to ask people to move, especially when the passengers are trying to avoid eye contact and your symptoms are invisible to them. For those using wheel-chairs, it can cause discomfort when the bus driver has to stop the bus and lower the lift, especially during busy times. A group member said that people often say, 'Can't you take another bus? We're trying to get to work on time.' This is especially hurtful when it has already taken a great deal of effort to get out of bed and get ready for the day.

Another member shared her disappointment with the group about being unable to attend a funeral because the other people she was planning to go with were taking public transportation. Missing out on special events and responsibilities can be distressing, especially when they are events that only occur once.

The fear of falling can also make travelling much more stressful. The group talked about how they have fallen in a variety of different places and how they have to worry about the possibility of not being able to get up.

Suggestions: Group members who use Dial-a-Ride/Access-a-Ride said that it is somewhat comforting to them because they don't have to worry about broken lifts/elevators in the underground/subway or jamming into crowded underground/subway coaches or buses during rush hour. Though it can be frustrating to deal with scheduling pick ups and drop offs, it tends to be a better option than the underground/subways or cancelling plans. Another group member addressed the issue of asking people to give up their seat on the bus. The group member encouraged the group to tell the driver that they needed a seat. It's the driver's responsibility to ask passengers to move if they do not have a medical reason for sitting.

It can be helpful to think of responses to rude passengers that can address their comments while also informing them about conditions like myositis. Also, you can only focus on your own mood and the way you treat other people, so feeling good about yourself may make it easier to overcome rude comments from others.

To help deal with the anxiety of falling, one group member said she carried her stick/cane. Even though she didn't always need it, it could give her support if necessary and ease her worry about being bumped by someone on the underground/subway or bus. One group member said that she found it helpful to have separate walkers for indoor and outdoor use. The group also talked about having several sets of the same assistive devices, such as high chairs and arm extenders, so that they are available no matter where in the home a person is at any given time.

Taking Medications

Many different medications are prescribed for patients with myositis to treat symptoms of inflammation, pain, swelling and fatigue. To treat multiple symptoms, a combination of medications may be prescribed to the same person. A frustration for those taking many medications is swallowing so many pills on a daily basis, often several times a day. In addition, some group members take their regular daily vitamins, thus increasing the number of pills they take each day.

The fear of side effects and interactions between medications can also be quite stressful. When one medication causes side effects or is not proving to be effective, a doctor may change the prescription. It can be difficult to change prescriptions because you may worry that you will suffer from ill side effects. Though doctors are usually aware of the medications a person is taking, group members mentioned that they often worry about possible interactions between medications. One group member shared that she recently experienced negative side effects when she began taking a new medication that interacted with another prescription she was taking. Another group member talked about how she gained a lot of weight from prednisone and that it caused her to worry about the health risks of a heavier weight.

Suggestions: One group member carries around a card listing all of her prescriptions and vitamins. At doctor appointments, the card is a reminder for the patient and the doctor, especially since many patients visit a number of doctors. The group also discussed how alternative therapies, eating well and exercising may be helpful in improving how a person feels, while potentially diminishing the need for other medications. Though many medications list a host of side effects, the group acknowledged that it doesn't mean that you'll experience any of them. Each person reacts differently. The group discussed the importance of concentrating on one's own individual health and treatment plan, because it isn't beneficial to compare side effects or CPK levels.

Stressful events occur for most people everyday. It can be very helpful to learn and practice stress reduction techniques, whether it's a massage or a funny movie. Members from our group suggested reading in the park, listening to a relaxation/nature CD, taking leisurely walks along the river, tuning into classical radio stations and writing in a journal. You may never be able to fully eliminate stress in your life, but you can develop more effective ways to cope with it.

The Impact of Myositis on Relationships

Myositis not only affects the person diagnosed, it also impacts on the members of their support system and thus the relationships they have with one another. Some relationships may be strengthened with adversity, while others may be weakened. Living with myositis can also affect how a person builds new connections with people. Although each person's support system is unique, with a variety of people and different types of relationship styles, there are common relationship challenges that emerge when dealing with a rare, chronic condition like myositis.

Advice-giving

People with myositis often have to deal with others trying to give them advice on how they can overcome their symptoms. It can be frustrating because other people often have little or no knowledge of what myositis is really about. Other people mistakenly think that there are simple ways to relieve its symptoms. Friends and family often give well-meaning advice, but sometimes their advice may do more harm than good. People without knowledge of myositis often say:

- 'Just take vitamin pills.'
- 'Get more sleep at night.'
- 'Try a home remedy.'
- 'Exercise more.'
- Lift weights to build muscle.'

One group member said that a family member wanted her to do intensive exercise and did not seem to fully understand how myositis had affected her strength. For example, she couldn't lift weights. The group also talked about being confronted with the old sayings, 'No pain, no gain' and 'The more you work, the better you'll feel.' The group felt that they are the real experts on their condition and sometimes resented that others think they know more.

One group member said that she sometimes wished that her friends would just listen and say they understood how she felt, rather than try to give advice. She wanted her friends to know that they didn't have to feel like they should 'fix' her disease because that wasn't what she was looking for from friends and family. The group talked about how their doctors are the people they turned to for medical advice. One group member said that even doctors weren't always educated about myositis and that it could cause you to lose trust in them. At times, they felt very lonely in their disease.

Many group members expressed their appreciation for the Myositis Support Group (USA and UK) because they could share their experiences with others who truly understood what they were going through. Members provide helpful suggestions for coping, as well as real and practical solutions for the challenges they face.

Misperceptions

Other people often misunderstand what having myositis actually means. When telling others that you have myositis, they often want to know first if it is life threatening and then once they realize that it's not, they don't really know how to react. Some group members had the feeling that some people thought they should be grateful that myositis is not necessarily critical. However, the severity of illness is not always the only determining factor for how a person copes. The idea of severity is relative, and 'quality of life' can be just as, or even more, important.

Many people have misperceptions about the disease and often mistakenly think it is contagious. A group member shared how the term 'autoimmune' has led people to believe that the member had HIV. Someone in that person's community told a family member that the member 'looked really good for having HIV.' Other group members said that the same thing had happened to them. The group said they realized that people are often afraid of things they aren't familiar with. Although group members don't always enjoy answering a lot of questions, they worry that some people just make assumptions when they don't have the correct information. Sometimes the assumptions can be worse than the reality and may leave others without compassion.

Educating Others

When diagnosed with a disease like myositis, some people feel like they are suddenly placed in a role where they have to educate others not only about their own condition, but also about all autoimmune diseases and chronic conditions. One group member shared that a family member had a different disease but had been doing really well, and she felt like her family expected her to cope just as well. Just because both of their diseases were rheumatic and chronic, her family members didn't seem to recognize that their diseases are very different. This type of comparison can also happen in any relationship where someone knows another person dealing with an autoimmune disease, rheumatic condition or other chronic illness.

Showing Emotion

People with rare diseases often struggle to help other people understand the realities of how their disease has affected them, because at the same time they are trying to avoid having their friends feel sorry for them. This is especially difficult when symptoms are invisible, like many of the symptoms of myositis. One group member said that her son's girl-friend was suspicious of her illness and almost believed that she was fak-ing her symptoms or making them seem worse than they really were. On the other hand, group members said that sometimes they felt like hiding their discomfort or weakness and wanted to portray themselves as feel-ing great. A person with myositis may try to cover up their feelings by:

- Putting on a happy face.
- Wearing their favourite clothes.
- Applying extra makeup and lipstick.
- Avoid talking about their symptoms.

Also, the group talked about how they didn't want others to feel like they are always talking about myositis. Sometimes they wanted to forget about their illness for awhile. When one group member reluctantly had to stop working, she was surprised by a co-worker's reaction of, 'Wow, you're not depressed.' Although this member really didn't feel all that great and was upset about quitting her job, she was also happy to catch up with her friend and had many good things in her life to focus on.

The group discussed the vulnerabilities of having a rare illness that people aren't educated about and how people often fear the unknown. One group member pointed out that she found herself being hesitant to become involved in new relationships, both romantic and friendly, because she feared having the other person reject her at some point in the future. She recognized that she was more protective of herself since she was diagnosed with myositis.

Recognising Physical Changes
Another complication of helping others understand myositis is that people with the disease themselves say that it can be hard for them to accept how myositis has caused changes in their bodies. Group mem-bers shared that sometimes they tried to push themselves to do things that they just weren't capable of doing anymore. A person who isn't ready to accept their limitations may:

- Continue at a job when unable to perform most duties.
- Overexert themselves going about their day as usual.

- Will themselves to do things like get out of a chair or climb stairs.
- Refuse to accept help when they really need it.

The group discussed how sometimes it takes other people to begin noticing their limitations in order for members to begin recognizing the symptoms themselves. It can be difficult to know how to talk to others about myositis when someone doesn't want to admit to himself that he has a disease. One member said he preferred to call it a 'condition', and many other group members agreed that this term is more comfortable for them to use when describing myositis. It can be scary not knowing what myositis really means, but it can also be scary to know a lot of information about it.

Stressing the importance of planning ahead

Living with a disease like myositis requires individuals to learn how to navigate a number of systems. The group expressed how they are still learning how to manoeuvre the city, with group members talking about their first ride on the city bus and trip to the cinema/movie or theatre. Group members talked about how they often had to plan ahead before going anywhere to make sure their entire trip was accessible. Planning ahead can be very time-consuming with many phone calls. It can involve a lot of extra steps, such as:

- Looking into various transportation options.
- Making sure that the destination doesn't have too many stairs.
- Figuring out if once they are inside, their wheelchair or walker will fit.
- Finding out whether or not the toilets/restrooms are accessible.

Although you may know how much effort is involved in checking the accessibility of a place, your friends and family may not. The group talked about how they are often invited out to dinner but then cannot attend because the restaurant is not accessible to them. One group member shared how she was so excited about her invitation to an open house for her nephew but when she realized his new apartment was up three storeys, she was really disappointed to have to decline the invite. The group talked about how having myositis makes them feel left out at times. They also said that they wouldn't want everyone to feel like everything always revolved around them. Rather than waiting for others to make plans or to wish they would consider your limitations when making plans, it might ease some frustration and disappointment to take on the role of the planner.

Asking for help

The group talked about how members of their support system often were well-meaning in their offer to help out, but that it could feel awkward to ask them for something when the need arose. Most group members have heard friends say, 'Let me know if you ever need me to get you anything at the supermarket.' However, one group expressed appreciation for friends who call to ask, 'Do you need anything from the supermarket because I'm on my way there?' The group agreed that this was a much more helpful question to ask and that they would feel more comfortable taking them up on it if the friend was offering to help at that moment. The group thought about how they could let their friends know what would be most helpful for them.

It can be frustrating when the people you deal with most on a daily basis don't do what you wish they would. The group discussed how they could use a different kind of help from significant others. At times, significant others can seem almost over-caring and members shared how they don't like being treated like a child. One group member said that even when completing a task that had resulted in a bad experience in the past, his significant other was surprised to find that he still wanted to try again. The group discussed how they didn't like others to just assume that they could never do that particular task ever again. One group member talked about how she had learned subtle ways to ask for help from her husband so that she didn't have to feel like she was always nagging him. People may feel that asking for help is bothersome and they should take pride in their independence. One group member added that he didn't like to ask for help with little things because his wife took care of so many bigger things. He really wished though that she would notice that she could help out with some more minor things as well.

The group also discussed how the need to use a wheelchair, walker or stick/cane leaves them feeling more vulnerable because there are times when they need to ask for help that involves physical contact. When a person needs to ask for physical help, they may worry about:

- Attracting attention from strangers.
- Having strangers or even their friends touch them.

- Feeling embarrassed.
- Falling.

Another relationship the group discussed was that of a parent and child and what it feels like to ask your child for help. Though the parent-child relationship naturally goes through a number of stages, when a parent is diagnosed with a disease like myositis with debilitating symptoms, it can accelerate the movement from one stage to another. Group members discussed their worry about burdening their children with the responsibility of caring for them if necessary. They also said they felt bad putting their children in the position of making a decision about whether or not they could care for their parent. The group pointed out that it almost seemed more unfair to care for a parent when it happened due to an illness rather than old age, even if both are occurring at the same time.

Lifestyle changes

When relationships revolve around a common interest in a particular activity, such as travelling, hiking, performing a job function or exercising, the interactions with these people can change after myositis. The group discussed how they felt like they have less in common with some of their friends, co-workers, neighbours, or even family members since myositis. Relationships may change because of the challenges of dealing with symptoms, such as:

- Cancelling plans at the last minute because you aren't feeling well.
- Physical limitations that keep you from pursuing prior interests.
- Preventing spontaneity in trying new activities or taking a trip.

A person with myositis may worry that others perceive them as unreliable when they cancel plans. They also worry that people may not want to share the details of an exciting trip or reaching a goal because the friend fears it might upset them. Not only do members miss the activities that once brought them great joy, they also miss the friendships. Though some friendships have changed and others have ended, there are people with common interests out there who are willing to make new friends. You can even find another friend dealing with myositis or a different chronic illness who can truly understand what it's like to experience it.

Coping with Myositis during the Holidays

Most of the time, the holidays are marked by joy and celebration. It is the season for giving and it generally puts people in a good mood. Yet, for people dealing with a chronic condition like myositis, the holidays can also bring a great deal of stress and frustration. Many of the holiday traditions of our group members have changed because of their fatigue, pain and limited mobility. Though they look forward to the excitement that the holidays bring, they have to adapt to doing things in a different way to take their symptoms of myositis into account.

The following describes challenges posed by different holiday traditions as well as helpful tips offered by our Myositis Support Group members:

1. Holiday celebrations often involve exchanging gifts.
Unfortunately, the act of shopping can present many obstacles for those dealing with myositis:

- Transportation to the stores.
- Carrying shopping bags.
- Manoeuvering around other shoppers.
- Cold and snowy December weather.

One member talked about learning to shop on the internet to have purchases delivered directly to the home of the person receiving the gift. Another group member mentioned finding a present that could be given to several people in order to cut down on the amount of time spent searching for individual gifts.

2. The holiday season also brings invitations to holiday parties.
Group members talked about how they are often invited to holiday parties by their workplace, spouses, families, children, friends or neighbourhood. At these parties, most people are not aware of the myositis, especially when symptoms aren't visible. At such, most guests stand, which can be difficult for people with myositis who need to sit down and rest for a bit. Sitting at a party can cause a person to feel:

- Left out of conversations.
- Worried that they are perceived as unsociable or lazy.

- Afraid that others will see them struggling to rise out of the chair.
- Viewed as not enjoying the party.

The group also talked about what it's like to use a wheelchair, walker, or stick/cane at a party. The group shared that, at times, the increased visibility can make it somewhat easier because others understand the person's difficulty in navigating the room and may make a point to come over. However, when holiday parties are held in locations with little space to move around, it can be frustrating to sit in one place all night and be dependent on others to take the initiative to come over and chat.

Using an assistive device to move around can also pose a challenge to holding a plate of food or grabbing a drink. This also adds to a feeling of dependency, especially when there's a need to ask strangers for help. An additional concern for users of wheelchairs and walkers is that the host of the party might experience it as a burden, especially if they need to make adjustments to the room or tend to the person during the party.

If you use a wheelchair, it was suggested that you let other party guests know that you would prefer to have them sit next to you, rather than stand over you. You can ask your host to help with introductions. When someone is getting a drink refilled, you can ask if they can get one for you also. This is a common request and wouldn't necessarily be viewed as dependency. It is important to find ways to assert yourself. Smiling, laughing, and conversing with others will help others notice that you're enjoying yourself and will draw them to you, even if you're not able to easily circulate around the room.

3. The holidays often involve eating many delicious (and tempting) foods.

Group members discussed their feelings about saying 'no' to sweets/puddings and alcohol because they want to avoid weight gain and have been told by their doctors to avoid alcohol. Sometimes, group members decide not to eat certain foods because they are unsure whether or not they will cause side effects with their medications. The group talked about whether or not they would be able to share a toast on New Year's Eve.

One group member said that one of her favourite parts of the holidays used to be cooking, but now she has difficulty carrying pots and pans and shopping for groceries. Another group member said that she used to host her entire family every year and would spend a lot of time decorating the house and cooking their favourite dishes. With myositis tiring her so easily, she is sad that she is no longer able to host the holidays.

The group talked about the time it takes to adjust to these new traditions and to accept their individual limitations. While this is often challenging, it is important to keep in mind that there are many ways to participate in the holidays and the new traditions might even end up being more fun and exciting than the old ones.

4. Many people create memories through traditional holiday activities.

New York City has a lot of holiday attractions that many group members remember fondly as part of their traditional holiday celebrations. Visiting the tree in Rockefeller Center, watching the holiday show at Radio City Music Hall, ice skating in Central Park, looking at the windows at Saks Fifth Avenue, and shopping are all fun holiday activities. However, they all require extra physical exertion, which can be difficult for people with myositis. These activities often present such challenges as:

- Walking long distances.
- Moving quickly with the flow of people.
- Waiting in long lines.
- Climbing theatre steps.
- Manoeuvering through large crowds.
- Withstanding cold weather.

Group members mentioned that the fatigue associated with myositis often makes these activities very difficult. They felt sad having to miss the activities they had once enjoyed and felt excluded when those around them continued to take part in these activities. The group thought it could be beneficial to find new places to visit in the holidays and considered that they might need to be the ones to organize the outing for their family or group of friends.

5. The holidays often mark the beginning of winter weather.
Having a disease that affects mobility can make a person more susceptible to inclement weather, which can also impact holiday celebrations.
One group member mentioned how much extra planning it took just
to go outside the house in the winter. She said that dressing herself
with extra layers took longer and sometimes she needed to make sure
that someone would be around to help her get ready. Another group
member said that she was most nervous about icy pavements/side-
walks and curbs. Getting around was already difficult with a stick/cane,
walker or wheelchair; cold, icy weather made it worse.

Winter weather can also cause isolation for people with myositis
who face challenges when travelling outdoors. Since leaving the house
takes a lot of energy and planning, group members shared that it was
often easier to stay at home. However, being stuck inside can create
feelings of depression. The group said that they find films/movies and
television helpful in keeping them entertained. Another member
encouraged the group to find a hobby, such as an arts and crafts project, to give them a goal to accomplish.

The holiday season is often a good time to reflect on your life and
the many changes you've gone through. It can be beneficial to spend
some time setting goals for the upcoming year.

*Angela Hunter, LMSW, coordinates a free monthly Myositis Support
Group, offered as a community service by Hospital for Special
Surgery's Department of Patient Care and Quality Management and
the Rheumatology Division. Ongoing since 1997, group meetings
include guest speakers and open discussions for people with myositis
and their families and friends. Additional summaries of selected
meetings are available at* www.hss.edu. *Ms. Hunter also works as a
program coordinator for international adoptions at Spence-Chapin
Services to Families and Children in New York City.*

8

When the Illness
is Invisible

by Lisa Copen

"But you look so good!"

"I can tell you must be feeling better. You look great!"

"I'm so glad you were able to come. Thank goodness you are finally getting some relief."

To a healthy person, none of these comments seem unusual or insincere. Our friends are simply trying to find the right thing to say. Of course, they really do believe that you must be feeling better or you wouldn't be out of bed. Those of us who are ill, however, understand that if we stayed in bed until we felt better, we would never leave the bedroom and we would miss out on life. So we get out of bed. We put our energy into finding something to wear that doesn't clash too badly; something that looks acceptable, despite the wrinkles. We search for the lipstick that we used last week. We dig through the wardrobe/closet looking for something that resembles a shoe. And we go on. We go out.

"But You Look So Good!"
Once we are out and about, people assume that we woke up feeling wonderful, that we jumped out of bed and are without pain. Says Donoghue and Siegel, authors of '*Sick and Tired of Feeling Sick and Tired*', "An added difficulty in adjusting to being handicapped with invisible chronic illness (ICI) is the phenomenon of appearing well."

Sometimes We Want to Appear Normal
Many chronic illnesses are invisible, causing feelings and frustrations that are different than what a person with a visible condition may expe-

rience. "It seems that we all want to appear normal. We all want to give the impression of strength, health and vigor," shares Camille Lewis, a graduate student at Indiana University who lives with Cushing's syndrome. "I've debated and debated about getting some walking help – a walking-stick/cane or whatever – and the one thing holding me back is my ego. I don't want to appear to be in pain. I want to be normal, even though I'm not."

Sometimes We Want People to Acknowledge the Pain

One would believe that pain would be socially understood and somewhat sympathized with. Although people do sympathize with pain, it is under circumstances that we believe are severely painful, such as childbirth, trauma, late stages of cancer, etc. People cannot relate with the chronically ill, since the individual is not screaming, crying or grimacing. We, who live with chronic pain, often walk, talk and function normally (as far as can be seen) so it is assumed that the pain is overstated. Migraines, for example, are often misunderstood as being just a bad headache.

Men who live with illnesses, such as fibromyalgia, may feel self-conscious. Their illness is primarily seen as a women's disease. They appear to be sluggish and unmotivated when they can't do physical tasks. Women are being diagnosed with chronic fatigue syndrome in huge numbers and yet the illness is still called "yuppie flu" and treated with anti-depressants. The immense fatigue that one suffers from is rarely recognized or understood by their friends and family around them.

We want People to Assume it's Just as Bad as it is, but No Worse than it Is

Living with an invisible chronic illness can mean constantly trying to redefine your condition. We can't keep up with the rest of the world and yet the world sees no excuse for our lack of participation. Some would argue that having an invisible chronic illness could be a blessing, as one has a choice to tell others or remain an assumed normal person. The disadvantage of this is trying to convince others that the disease is legitimate and painful. Many people think "Aren't you overdoing it... or playing it up a little bit?" People's observations do not conform to their expectations as to what a sick person should look and act like. Therefore, they are quick to become intolerant and suspect that the symptoms are overstated. It is often not only the disease itself that is painful, but also the emotional effects of having the illness discounted, having one's respectability and judgment questioned and dealing with the criticisms of others. It is extremely necessary for the person with chronic illness to feel that his disease is validated, even by people that he doesn't know. One example of this is "the handicapped parking space confrontation."

The Need to Feel Validated
There are over 40 million people who live with chronic illness in the United States, most of the illnesses are invisible. Often, illnesses make it difficult for the person to walk far and so handicapped placards are issued to them. The placard holders are soon often confronted by accusatory looks, stares, notes left on their windscreen/windshield and even approached and questioned about their obvious lack of wheelchair. For those who have experienced any one of these situations, it can be a humiliating and frustrating situation. None of us feel as though we should have to justify our illness to anyone and yet we are so angered by their obvious ignorance and their belief that we are abusing the "privilege" (that we wish we weren't applicable to receive). Although they are complete strangers, we still have a desire for their understanding and validation.

What to do?
So what do we do with these frustrations and the lack of understanding that we may sometimes feel that other people have? David Biebel, author of *If God Is So Good Why Do I Hurt So Bad?* writes in his book, "Because God is now here, I am not an only child. I have a friend, closer than a brother, who understands the path I walk because He has walked it too. His heart beats with mine. His heart breaks with mine. His hands reach out, through their own pain, to touch my aching soul and let me know that someday it will all become clear – but for now to keep on walking, like He did and like others have before me"

Lisa Copen is the founder and director of Rest Ministries. She lives with rheumatoid arthritis and fibromyalgia and is the author of When Chronic Illness Enters Your Life Bible Study.
Reprinted from ...And He Will Give You Rest
monthly support newsletter, Volume 11, Issue 3. © *1998.*

9

Counselling and Myositis

by William West BSc., MA., PhD., Fellow BACP
Senior Lecturer in Counselling Studies,
University of Manchester

What is counselling?

According to the British Association for Counselling and Psychotherapy (1997) counselling is defined as:

> *'to provide an opportunity for the client to work towards living in a way he or she experiences as more satisfying and resourceful. The term 'counselling' includes work with individuals, pairs or groups of people often, but not always referred to as 'clients'. The objectives of particular counselling relationships will vary according to the client's needs. Counselling may be concerned with developmental issues, addressing and resolving specific problems, making decisions, coping with crisis, developing personal insight and knowledge, working through feelings of inner conflict or improving relationships with others. The counsellor's role is to facilitate the client's work in ways that respect the client's values, personal resources and capacity for choice within his or her cultural context.*
>
> *Counselling involves a deliberately undertaken contract with clearly agreed boundaries and commitment to privacy and confidentiality. It requires explicit and informed agreement.'*

It should be clear from the above definition of counselling how potentially useful it can be for any one of us at difficult moments in our lives. The value of seeing a counsellor rather than close friends or family is that the counsellor is uninvolved in our lives, has no axe to grind and should possess some considerable experience and training in working with people facing the common issues and problems in living. Counsellors are not intended to take the place of good friends and family.

How to find a counsellor?

Over half the GP surgeries in Britain now have counsellors. Those that do not should be able to make an appropriate referral as should most consultants. Counselling is provided by trained counsellors who are often accredited by the British Association for Counselling and Psychotherapy, or by counselling psychologists registered with the British Psychological Society and increasingly by Community Psychiatric Nurses. There are also a number of excellent voluntary agencies providing counselling sometimes to particular groups e.g. Relate (for relationships), Victim Support (for crime victims), Cruse (for the bereaved) and many churches and other religious groups have counselling services. Local voluntary groups can be contacted via the local Citizens Advice Bureau. For those willing to pay for counselling the British Association for Counselling and Psychotherapy can be contacted, phone 0870 443 5252 or web site: *www.bacp.co.uk*. If it is clear to your GP or your counsellor that you need to work therapeutically at a deeper level you will likely be recommended for psychotherapy.

What is counselling like?

Seeing a counsellor is very different from seeing your GP or other health professional. For a start most counsellors will book you in for at least 50 minutes and will aim to be free to see you at the fixed appointment time. You are likely to have several sessions with your counsellor. Merely having such a period of time in which the counselling will focus on you and your problems is a very unusual experience for most of us. It can be a very healing time. You will be invited to set the agenda for the counselling and your counsellor will probably not give you any direct advice on what to do. The idea of counselling is to help you figure out for yourself what is best for you, help you explore the difficulties you are experiencing.

What kind of counselling is best for people who live with myositis?

There are a number of different counselling approaches some of which you may have heard of, or come across, including person-centred, psychodynamic, cognitive-behavioural and integrative. There has been much research and debate into which counselling approach works best with which problem. However, the research tends to show that there is little to choose between the different approaches and that good counselling depends on a good relationship between counsellor and client. The best counsellors are those who you trust, feel listened by, and who feel helpful to you.

How can counselling benefit people living with myositis?

Whenever people who have received counselling for almost any condition or problem are asked whether it helped them, invariably 4 out of 5 reply it was helpful or very helpful. It is highly unlikely that counselling can 'cure' myositis. However, we do know that the mind can affect the body (and vice versa) and that emotional and psychological states can affect the functioning of the body's immune system. Dealing with what might be a long term and unpredictable illness like myositis is best done from a position of psychological and emotional strength which is where counselling comes in.

According to the Myositis Support Group UK website, following a diagnosis of myositis 'depression and a general feeling of misery can frequently ensue'. This is where counselling or some other form of psychological help and support is vital. The website also states 'for the majority it is a case of coping with the disease and trying to live as near a normal life as possible'. The challenge of coping with myositis is often met with support from family and friends. However, family and friends are at the same time having to face the changes wrought in their lives by the illness of their loved ones. Support by others with myositis can be a key factor in facing the illness and counselling can play its part both for the patient and those close to them.

As will be apparent from the other chapters in this book, the time before a diagnosis of myositis is made can itself be a time of great stress and confusion. Whilst the diagnosis itself might produce some feelings of relief it will likely necessitate considerable change and adjustment to both the individual and their family. The impact on the family and close friends might well get in the way of the usual support systems in place for the person living with the illness. Likewise a stay in hospital can weaken such support. Counselling can clearly help in these early stages pre and post diagnosis.

Since the unfolding of the illness can itself be unpredictable there may well be times when counselling becomes once more useful. It is not only bad news that is difficult to hear and deal with. Remission or even the cure of an illness can also prove troublesome. All involved could have got use to, and adjusted to, the limitations imposed by an illness at one point in time only to have the whole picture confounded.

Will my counsellor know about my illness?

Since it is a relatively rare illness it is unlikely that your counsellor will know much about myositis. Your counsellor should have some under-standing of living with chronic illness and the kind of problems that might ensue. Nevertheless the counsellor will consider you to be the 'expert' in your illness and will listen carefully to your experience of liv-ing with myositis. Do not be afraid of 'educating' your counsellor about your illness. Having heard from you about myositis (or your GP when she or he refers you to the counsellor) it is probable that your counsel-lor will then seek out useful information about it from a number of sources in order to help you in the most beneficial way.

Conclusion

Counselling is a human activity undertaken by one human with another, with a couple or with a group. Experienced counsellors will have faced the whole range of human experience from relationship break up, sex-ual abuse, alcohol and drug addiction, death, mid life crisis, loneliness as well as more specifically illness related problems. However counsel-lors are not just there for major problems – no issue should be seen as being too small. If you are sufficiently troubled by something then con-sider counselling. Sometimes even a good happy life can be problem-atic – we can be haunted by fears that it will all go wrong so that we are unable to enjoy our good fortune. Counselling then can have a use to others living with myositis. It is not a panacea but nevertheless can be of great help to most of those who seek its services.

William West works full-time as the Director of Counselling Courses at the University of Manchester. He is a Fellow, accredited counsellor and Special Adviser on Research to the British Association for Counselling and Psychotherapy. His first book 'Psychotherapy and Spirituality' was published by Sage in January 2000 and his second book 'Spiritual Issues in Therapy' was published by Palgrave Macmillan in 2003. William lives in Manchester with his wife and young daughter.

SECTION THREE

Therapies

10

Current
Treatment

by Dr Rob Fenton, BSc (Hons) PhD

I have listed below the standard treatment for myositis, experimental treatment and other treatment which has been tried in a limited way but has not proved useful. I have used some generic names and some product names. Some treatments are better for one type of myositis than another, and not all treatments give benefit to all types of myositis.

Often treatment is given as combinations e.g. a steroid coupled with a non-steroidal immunosuppressive.

I have included some additional/supplementary treatments used to treat side effects of medication e.g. to stop bone loss (osteoporosis) in patients taking corticosteroids (steroids), or to alleviate symptoms of the disease. This list is not meant to be exhaustive and I apologise to any manufacturer whose product is not represented here.

Inclusion body myositis (IBM) is particularly difficult to treat, although a few patients do respond to some extent to some of the drugs listed below.

Current Approaches

The standard treatment in the UK is high-dose oral prednisolone (sometimes preceded by three intravenous doses of methylprednisolone in severe disease). Combination therapies with immunosuppressants and steroids will allow more rapid reduction of the steroid dose. Cytotoxics of first choice are methotrexate and azathioprine, with cyclophosphamide or chlorambucil reserved for severe disease which is unresponsive to first line therapy, or when there is severe internal organ involvement such as pulmonary fibrosis.

Mycophenolate is a newer option and IVIg is another therapy (previously used in vasculitis).

• **Immunosuppressants** – These include prednisolone/prednisone and methylprednisolone (all three are corticosteroids, prednisone being a synthetic prodrug that is converted by the liver into prednisolone, which is the active drug; prednisolone is prescribed in the UK, whilst prednisone is prescribed in the USA), Maxtrex or Rheumatrex (methotrexate), Imuran (azathioprine), Neoral/SangCya/Sandimmune (cyclosporin), Cytoxan (cyclophosphamide), Cellcept (mycophenolate mofetil), Prograf (tacrolimus, FK506) etc. All of these treatments suppress the normal immune responses (reducing the activity and proliferation of immune cells such as lymphocytes), which in the case of myositis sufferers are thought to be inappropriately damaging normal muscle tissue. Prednisolone/prednisone is used as a first-line treatment. If the patient does not improve after a short period, or has a flare whenever prednisolone is tapered, then methotrexate or sometimes azathioprine is used as second-line therapy in combination with the steroid. In patients who do not respond to either corticosteroids or second-line agents then there are several third-line agents (e.g. cyclosporin, cyclophosphamide) which are available. These drugs are more toxic than steroids or second-line agents and so have to be monitored carefully.

• **Prednisolone** – In acute myositis the starting dosage is frequently high (~40-60mg per day) tapering down with time over months, if not years. Prednisone needs conversion in the liver to become active, and so higher doses may need to be used in patients with liver disease (e.g. hepatitis, cirrhosis). Patients taking prednisolone or prednisone should never suddenly stop taking the treatment as this could prove dangerous. This is because systemic steroids suppress the production of the body's natural corticosteroids (adrenal suppression) and the body needs time to recover In addition, discontinuing steroid use too abruptly can lead to a flare (rebound) of the disease and this would then require a return to the larger dose. You <u>must always</u> be guided by your doctor who will advise on schedules to help you reduce the dosage. Corticosteroids can cause calcium loss from the bones resulting in osteoporosis. Patients on long term, moderate or high dose treatment should be monitored with bone density scans, and will require calcium/vitamin D supplements and bone building treatments from a family of drugs called bisphosphonates (see below). Other steroid side effects may include 'moon-face', hair thinning, increased facial hair, skin thinning and scarring, spontaneous bruising, weight gain, bloating, mood swings, acne, gastrointestinal problems, increased appetite and poor sleep patterns. Prednisolone brand names include Orapred, Pediapred and Prelone. Brand names for prednisone include Deltasone, Meticorten, Orasone, Prednicen-M, and Sterapred. Methylprednisolone has the brand name Solumedrol. Patients on steroids should also have annual eye check-ups, as this treatment can also cause cataracts and raised intraocular pressure (glaucoma).

• **IVIG** – Intravenous immunoglobulin. IVIg has been used for decades in many different inflammatory diseases with an autoimmune component. It has some limited benefit and is often used when response to first-line therapy is poor. Normal antibodies extracted from pooled blood from donors can be given by an infusion (similar to a blood transfusion) which may be given over several days and then repeated months later. This is believed to suppress the function of abnormally active immune cells by binding to cell surface regulators. It works for immune mediated blood disorders and is a safe add-on therapy in myositis and lupus-like disorders. Indeed, this treatment has shown positive benefits to both dermatomyositis and polymyositis patients, in clinical trials. Side effects are common, but these are usually mild. They include headache, increased muscle pain (myalgia), nausea, vomiting, fatigue, fever, chills and low blood pressure (hypotension). These effects usually occur at the time of infusion.

Treatment in the experimental stage

• **Biologics**
Enbrel (etanercept) – This is available in the USA and the UK for the treatment of Rheumatoid Arthritis (RA). Enbrel is a synthetic protein consisting of the cell surface part of a natural receptor to human tumour necrosis factor (TNFR). This protein is linked to part of a synthetic human antibody. This biologically active agent inactivates Tumour Necrosis Factor Alpha (TNFα) by binding to it. TNFα is

thought to be a key inflammatory substance in rheumatoid arthritis and Enbrel has been of enormous benefit to many patients with this condition. Twice weekly subcutaneous injections are known to mop up excess TNFα and reduce inflammation. Experimentally, this drug has now been used to treat interstitial pulmonary fibrosis (IPF) i.e. where there is lung involvement, a condition <u>sometimes</u> associated with myositis. The problem with this and similar anti-cytokine directed treatments, is that patients can develop severe infections, and rare cases of developing autoimmune disease have been reported. It remains an experimental therapy for myositis.

Remicade (infliximab) – This is a human/mouse IgG(1) kappa mono-clonal antibody acting directly against TNFα molecules which are key in the production of inflammation. At the time of writing, clinical trials are underway to determine the effectiveness of this treatment in der-matomyositis and polymyositis patients. One disadvantage of inflix-imab is that it requires 6-8 weekly visits to hospital for a slow intravenous infusion.

Rituxan (rituximab) – This is an anti-B lymphocyte agent (monoclon-al antibody to B cells). B lymphocytes are the white blood cells respon-sible for producing antibodies which normally neutralise viral and bacterial infections. In myositis, B lymphocytes may inappropriately produce antibodies against self-proteins and either directly or indi-rectly damage tissues. Treatment with this agent is by infusion (usually 2 doses two weeks apart). In patients with rheumatoid arthritis, clini-cal benefit takes a few weeks to occur but can then last for months or even years. At the time of writing, a pilot study of Rituxan in patients with DM in the USA looks very promising.

Eculizumab – This is another humanised monoclonal antibody, which attacks C5 complement. C5 complement acts in conjunction with autoantibodies to attack the muscle cells, in myositis conditions. This treatment has given mixed results in clinical trials with rheumatoid arthritis patients, but has been studied in DM patients with some improvements observed, in particular a reduction in the associated skin rashes.

Campath (alemtuzumab) – Campath is also a humanised monoclonal antibody. It is currently approved to treat certain leukaemias, but has been used against some autoimmune conditions (e.g. vasculitis, multiple sclerosis, rheumatoid arthritis) and also to reduce tissue rejection associated with transplantation. Campath destroys T lymphocytes that have a protein called CD52 on their surface. These lymphocytes are one of the cell types responsible for damaging muscle in myositis patients. Other white blood cells expressing CD52 are monocytes, macrophages and monocyte-derived dendritic cells. These may also be suppressed by Campath playing a role in reducing inflammation. This treatment is currently being assessed in IBM patients to see if it improves muscle strength.

Antegren – Yet another monoclonal antibody. These antibodies target areas (receptors) on the surface of white blood cells (lymphocytes), rendering them incapable of migrating to sites of inflammation and causing further damage to the tissues they are programmed to attack.   The receptors in question are known as alpha-4-beta-1 (VLA-4) and alpha-4-beta-7 integrins. These antibodies may be useful for any inflammatory disease, and it is already known that lymphocytes present in the muscles of polymyositis and dermatomyositis express VLA-4 receptors. To date, the author knows of no myositis patient to be treated by this approach.

Avonex – This beta interferon 1a has been shown to have a beneficial effect in Multiple Sclerosis (MS) patients. A pilot study in IBM patients showed no effect, though at the time of writing, further trials with higher doses are ongoing.

The following drugs have been tried in a limited way to treat myositis and have shown some benefit in a few cases. However, it is unlikely that they will be subjected to further trials in the future.

• **Leukeran** (chlorambucil) – Leukeran is normally given as a treatment for cancer. It has been shown to be beneficial in treating leukaemias and some lymphomas. Because it is effective in eliminating white cells (T and B cells), it has been suggested that it may have use in treating myositis. In a very small group of dermatomyositis patients, which had previously shown to be resistant to steroid, azathioprine and methotrexate treatment, this drug was shown to have some benefit. However, as with most anti-cancer treatments, there are significant side effects. The most important of these is that Leukeran itself increases the risk of new cancers. In addition, it can have profound effects on fertility in both men and women, and it should be avoided during pregnancy. In short term usage, there is an increased risk of infection, and nausea and vomiting are common.

• **Hydroxychloroquine sulphate** (Plaquenil) – This is used primarily for malaria, but has been shown to benefit patients with SLE (systemic lupus erythematosus) and rheumatoid arthritis (which are also autoimmune diseases). This drug may also benefit patients with myositis, but as yet the information available is limited. However, it does appear to be effective in treating the persistent rashes associated with both adult and juvenile dermatomyositis. It may reduce cholesterol levels for patients on prednisolone.

• **Fludara** (fludarabine) – As with chlorambucil, this drug is normally given as an anti-cancer agent, most commonly used to treat chronic lymphocytic leukaemia. Side effects are likely to be similar to those mentioned for chlorambucil. In a limited clinical trial of 16 patients with either DM or PM, whose previous treatments had proven ineffective, only 4 patients showed improvement of their condition.

• **Minocin/Dynacin/Vectrin** (minocycline) is a derivative of the antibiotic tetracycline. It has been used in rheumatoid arthritis with limited success and has been suggested as a treatment for systemic lupus erythematosus (SLE). However, it has also been shown to induce a Lupus syndrome, inflammatory arthritis, skin rashes, and autoimmune hepatitis. The use of this treatment for myositis is yet to be proven.

• **Arava** (leflunomide) – This medication is classified as a disease-modifying anti-rheumatic drug (DMARD), which helps improve RA symptoms such as joint swelling and tenderness. This agent has been used in myositis patients off label, but little information is available.

• **Dapsone** – An anti-leprosy/anti-malarial treatment that may have limited benefit in myositis patients, because of its efficacy in vasculitis.

Additional/supplementary treatments

These are treatments which are not used to treat myositis per se but are used to treat side effects of medication or to alleviate symptoms of the disease.

- **NSAIDs** (**N**on **S**teroidal **A**nti-**I**nflammatory **D**rugs) These drugs, as a group, are effective for pain relief and may also be used for their anti inflammatory action in myositis patients. Some NSAIDs are thought to block platelet over-activity in the blood. Low dose aspirin can be used for this very reason, on an empirical basis, as the vessel wall and platelet interaction can be part of the disease damage in myositis. Stomach pains (due to gastritis and rare instances of bleeding ulcers), fluid retention and kidney damage can be as a consequence of these drugs, which should always be taken with physician's advice when patients have a complex disease such as myositis. Examples of NSAIDs are: Naprosyn/Arthrosin/Synflex/Timpron (naproxen), Diclofenac and Indomethacin. (N.B. Ibuprofen and newer agents such as Rofecoxib, Celecoxib and Etoricoxib have short lasting effects or minimal action on platelets, so the choice of agent may be important.) This whole group of drugs are currently under scrutiny because of a recently noted increase in heart attacks and strokes.

- **Biophosphonates** are drugs which inhibit bone resorption (break down) e.g. Fosamax (alendronate), Didronel PMO (etidronate disodium), Aredia (pamidronate), Actonel (risedronate), Zometa (zoledronate) and Boniva (ibandronate). Patients who take steroids such as prednisolone, prednisone or dexamethasone for long periods almost always have decreased bone density and may be at increased risk of breaking a bone. Both treatments are taken along with calcium (e.g. Calcichew) and vitamin D supplements. Research has shown that pamidronate also improves bone density in adults who take glucocorticoids, but this involves an intravenous infusion (i.e. a drip in hospital). However, use of pamidronate is not yet approved in children.

- **Potassium** supplements (e.g. SLOW-K, SANDO-K). Corticosteroids can occasionally cause a reduction in blood potassium levels.

- **Creating supplements** Creatine has been used by athletes to improve muscle strength, when combined with exercise. Recent clinical trials showed that in myositis patients, creatine with exercise improved muscle strength by approximately 10% after 6 months. This improvement was similar to findings in normal untreated control patients on a similar exercise program, indicating that it is unclear whether the addition of creatine was of benefit or not.

• **Folicare, Lexpec, Preconcieve etc.** (folic acid) This is always given to patients undergoing treatment with methotrexate (an analogue of folic acid), to avoid the potential serious side effects of methotrexate induced folate deficiency.

Additional non-drug aspects of management

In addition to the 'standard drug treatment' of myositis, it is extremely important for the patient to seek advice on physiotherapy and exercise, occupational therapy, nutrition etc. Other chapters in this book will be a good starting point in education.

11
Nutrition

by Audrey Howe, BSc, D.N.Med

This chapter is written to provide general dietary guidelines on how to minimise the unwanted effects of steroids. We have put together frequently asked questions and given some very broad dietary steps that can be taken. However, to gain maximum advantage from your diet it is advisable to consult a nutritionist who can assess your individual needs.

These guidelines are very general and may not be appropriate for all.

How do I keep my blood sugar levels up without causing weight gain?

Weight gain associated with steroid use results partly from excessive lows in blood sugar, which leads to the need to eat frequently. If inappropriate foods are chosen difficulties with blood sugar control are exacerbated and weight gain continues.

Foods from which sugars are absorbed slowly into the bloodstream help maintain steady blood sugar levels.

Action:

1. Eat at least 3 meals per day, including breakfast soon after getting up. Don't attempt to miss meals in order to lose weight – it will only lead to snacking on sugary foods and drinks, or eating more later on in the day.

2. It might be useful to eat 4-6 smaller, more frequent meals, than the traditional three main meals (eating half quantities of each meal will save on time preparing these).

3. Avoid sugar and refined foods such as biscuits, cakes, white flour and white rice. These immediately raise blood sugar, but a sharp drop soon follows and with it a return to hunger or sugar cravings.

   Honey and dried fruits are often substituted for sugar and whilst these do make useful sweeteners, they should not be used in large quantities. Two teaspoons of honey or a small handful of dried fruit per day should be the maximum used.

   Also avoid artificial sweeteners, as these make the body think it is going to receive sugar, and increase sugar cravings.

4. Eat complex carbohydrates rather than simple sugars. This means avoiding sugary foods and drinks such as biscuits, sweets, fruit squashes, and canned drinks. Use instead whole grains such as brown rice, millet, potatoes in their skins or wholemeal bread.

5. To ensure that foods are absorbed slowly, include in each meal small amounts of protein and fat, although not too much as this can have a detrimental effect on digestion and health. This should be combined with some complex carbohydrate, and some vegetables. This sounds complicated, but in practise is quite simple, an example, is chicken and vegetable stir-fry served with brown rice and a small quantity of olive oil added to the dish on serving.

   100g of meat, 150g of fish, 2 eggs are appropriate serving sizes of protein for a main meal. Meals that do not contain meat, fish or eggs, should contain lentils, beans or nuts as protein sources.

   Olive oil or linseed oil may be added as dressing to give some beneficial fats. These should not cause weight gain, but rather are thought to assist in weight loss, through increased metabolism of fats.

6. Avoid tea and coffee. These have a similar effect to simple sugars, causing sudden increase in blood sugar, followed by a low.

7. Avoid low fat and diet foods.

8. Choose appropriate snacks – see below. You may need to keep one next to the bed in case blood sugar falls during the night.

9. A small snack before bed will help prevent blood sugar falling too low during the night. A small bowl of porridge, using oats and

water is useful, as the oats are also soothing to the nervous system and will help to give a good night's sleep.

What can I eat to avoid high blood pressure?

Foods rich in magnesium and potassium are very useful in keeping blood pressure down. Sodium and salty foods however are likely to raise blood pressure. The amount and type of fat in the diet also has a great impact on blood pressure.

Include

- *Magnesium rich foods:*
  Green leafy vegetables – kale, endive lettuce, watercress
  Pulses – mung beans, red lentils, chickpeas, butterbeans
  Seeds – sesame (tahini is a sesame spread), sunflower seeds
  Fruit

- *Potassium rich foods:*
  Green leafy vegetables as above
  Root vegetables – carrot, swede, turnip
  Celery
  Cauliflower
  Fruit

Vegetable intake is very important and a range of fresh vegetables should be included daily in as large a quantity as possible. Try to include a vegetable soup, a salad and some form of cooked vegetables.

- Garlic and onions, which have a known effect on lowering blood pressure. The effect is more pronounced if they are taken raw.

- 1-2 stalks of celery a day, as this is thought to have a particularly beneficial effect.

- Extra Virgin Olive oil and Linseed oils as salad dressings.

- Oily fish such as salmon, mackerel, sardine, trout, herring at least 3 times per week. Vary the types used.

- 1-2 litres of mineral or filtered water, per day.

Beware of

- Added salt and salty foods. Avoid adding salt to cooking or at the table, and avoid salty foods such as marmite, cheeses, instant potato mixes, sauce mixes, crisps, sausages, take-aways.

- Alcohol and coffee.

- High intakes of saturated fat such as those in butter and cream. Saturated fat occurs in high levels in cakes, pastry and biscuits.

- Red meat. Minimise intake, particularly of beef and pork.

- Vegetable oils such as sunflower oil, corn oil. These should not be used in cooking. Use only Extra Virgin Olive oil for any shallow frying, and fry slowly at low temperatures.

- Margarines and spreadable fats. If using fats for spreading, use either unsalted butter, in strict moderation, or non-hydrogenated margarines. A good variety is Vitaquel margarine, available from most health food shops.

How do I minimise fluid retention?

Follow the advice above for avoiding high blood pressure. Additionally carrot juice, cucumber, pear, radish and nettle tea may help reduce the amount of water in the body, without the disadvantage of potassium losses, which is common with diuretic drugs.

How do I minimise the risk of osteoporosis?

Calcium deficiency is generally associated with osteoporosis and milk and its products are thought of as good sources of this mineral. However, calcium from milk is not well absorbed or used by the body and can actually have an adverse effect upon osteoporosis. In addition, many people with an immune condition such as myositis also have food allergies, dairy being a common one.

Ensuring sufficient levels of other minerals such as magnesium, manganese and boron is also important in avoiding osteoporosis but these are often overlooked.

Include
- Calcium rich foods from non-dairy sources. Green vegetables are a source of calcium, which should not be under estimated. To illustrate this we must observe that cows living solely on green grasses produce calcium rich milk. Some rich vegetable sources of calcium are curly kale, watercress, broccoli, spring greens, carrot, turnip and swede.

  A diet built around cereals such as oats and brown rice, pulses, nuts and fruit and vegetables can provide a quite sufficient calcium intake. Canned fish eaten with the bones is also a very good source.

- Magnesium rich foods such as green leafy vegetables – kale, endive lettuce, watercress, Pulses – mung beans, red lentils, chickpeas, butterbeans, Seeds – sesame (tahini is a sesame spread), sunflower seeds, fruit

- Foods such as apples, pears, peaches, almonds and hazelnuts contain boron.

- Manganese rich foods such as nuts, oatmeal, pineapple, blackberries.

Beware of
- Tea and coffee. Both these tend to strip calcium from the bones.
- Fizzy drinks
- High alcohol intake.
- Salt and salty foods.
- High intakes of red meat, particularly beef and pork.
- Dairy products.

I get recurrent urinary tract infections; can I do anything to prevent this?

The health of the urinary tract is dependent upon the bacterial population there and this in turn is strongly influenced by intestinal bacteria. Billions of bacteria live in the intestinal tract. Some are beneficial and essential for health, others are considered non-beneficial, but these are usually kept under control by the beneficial species. Heavy doses of steroids disrupt the balance of these bacteria and predispose to conditions such as cystitis. The diet should therefore include foods that nourish the beneficial bacteria and avoid foods nourishing to the non-beneficial bacteria.

Include

- A high intake of vegetables. Again onion and garlic are very beneficial, but a wide variety of vegetables should be included.
- A good quality supplement of beneficial bacteria such as acidophilus or bifidus.
- Two litres of water daily.
- Cranberry juice – a chemical in this has been found to prevent infectious bacteria attaching to cells lining the urinary tract.
- Blueberries – have a similar effect to cranberries.

Beware of

- Sugar
- Alcohol
- Yeast and fermented foods
- Wheat
- Dairy
- High intakes of meat
- Caffeine

What can I eat instead?

If you are now wondering what you can possibly eat, be assured that there are many tasty alternatives.

Sufferers of auto-immune conditions often also experience food allergies. Wheat and dairy allergies are the most common and it is advisable to cut these out of the diet for a few weeks and see if you notice any improvement in the way you feel.

The table below gives some alternative to commonly eaten foods. Coeliacs and those who require gluten free diets can use rice, millet, buckwheat, polenta and quinoa but should avoid wheat, barley, oats and rye.

What I did eat	Substitutes
Bread	Rye bread or rye crackers such as Ryvita. Instead of sandwiches, make a rice salad.
Pasta	Non-wheat pastas e.g. corn pasta, buckwheat pasta. Use brown rice, jacket potato, millet, barley or buckwheat instead.
Flour	Non-wheat flours can be used in baking e.g. brown rice flour, chickpea flour.
Cereals such as Weetabix, Shredded Wheat	Porridge Wheat-free muesli Puffed rice pops (sugar free)
Biscuits	Unsalted Rice Cakes with a spread Low salt oat cakes Corn crackers
Milk	Soya milk Rice milk Oat milk Nut milk
Yoghurt	Sheep or goats yoghurt Soya yoghurt
Cheese	Tahini, houmous, nut butter
Tea	Fruit teas, herbal teas, Redbush tea
Coffee	Dandelion coffee, Barley cup, Caro (the latter two are not gluten free)
Fizzy Drinks	Water, diluted pure fruit juice

Menu building

Choose one item from each column,

Protein	Carbohydrate	Fat	
Fish – especially oily fish	Brown Rice Millet	Olive oil Linseed oil	**Vegetables in some form – soup, salad, steamed, casseroled, stir-fried**
Meat – most beneficial – poultry, lamb	Rye bread/Ryvita Wholemeal bread	Seeds Nuts	
Egg (organic)	Potato	Unsalted organic butter (very small quantities)	
Lentils	Polenta		
Beans	Corn crisp bread	Non-hydrogenated margarine	
Tofu	Buckwheat		
Nuts	Barley	Avocado	

Snacks

Unsalted rice cakes or oat cakes with tahini, avocado, houmous or nut butter
Fruit
Handful of nuts
Handful of seeds
Popcorn
Houmous and raw vegetable strips
Soya yoghurt

Example menus

Breakfast: Porridge (made with water or a non-dairy milk) + fruit/dried fruit if desired.

Mid morning: Rice Cakes and avocado

Lunch: Salmon sandwich (in wholewheat or rye bread)
Mid afternoon: Houmous and celery sticks
Dinner: Vegetable soup. Chicken stir-fry served with brown rice.

Breakfast: Scrambled egg on toast (wholewheat or rye)
Mid morning: Fruit
Lunch: Salad with steamed trout and quinoa
Mid afternoon: Oatcakes and tahini
Dinner: Lentil stew served with mashed potato and steamed vegetables

A gluten and dairy free menu
Breakfast: Porridge made from millet flakes and rice flakes and water or non-dairy milk + fruit or dried fruit if desired.
Mid morning: Rice cakes and almond butter or avocado
Lunch: Vegetable soup. Tuna salad and millet.
Mid afternoon: Fruit
Dinner: Lamb Curry served with brown rice and steamed vegetables

Breakfast: Egg fried rice.
Mid morning: Handful of nuts and seeds.
Lunch: Lentil soup. Jacket potato with mackerel and salad.
Mid afternoon: Soya yoghurt with fruit if desired.
Dinner: Bean and vegetable casserole with millet.

Audrey Howe graduated from the Plaskett Nutritional Medicine College in 1998 and now works as a nutritional therapist in West London and Oxfordshire.

Audrey Howe can be contacted at: -
http://www.nutrition.therapist.org.uk

12

The Role of an Occupational Therapist

by Julie Mallen, Dip. C.O.T., S.R.O.T.
Senior Occupational Therapist,
Devon Social Services

Editor's Note

Although this chapter sometimes talks about the more serious levels of disability, this will not necessarily apply to everyone. All conditions are different and bring a range of needs. Many people living with myositis may never need mechanical aids or occupational therapy equipment. Others might use them only when their illness is at its peak.

What is Occupational Therapy?

Occupational Therapy (O.T.), is a method of treatment to help people who are vulnerable or disabled. Therapists may work with children, people with learning disabilities, physical disabilities, or mental health problems. The aim of therapy is to restore or regain function in activities of daily living (occupations), to enable people to live more productive lives and to promote maximum independence.

The activities we all do everyday such as cooking, shopping, maintaining personal care, leisure interests, employment and so on, often need to be adapted in some way to enable those with disabilities to continue them. In many situations it is the person themselves who might need to learn adaptive techniques, or the environment which needs to be adapted.

To qualify as a therapist, students must complete at least a three-year course, which covers topics such as physiology, psychiatry, medicine, anatomy, child development, sociology, surgery, as well as theories in Occupational Therapy.

The role of an Occupational Therapist is diverse, and a qualified therapist may work within a hospital setting, rehabilitation centre, Social Services, client's home, private clinics, within day care/respite units, or a G.P. surgery. Many people will understand the role of a Physiotherapist, but it is no wonder the role of Occupational Therapy is difficult to appreciate when it fulfils so many functions and in so many different areas.

Occupational Therapists carry out an assessment of need, to establish the reasons why someone can no longer carry out everyday activities which, when we are well, take for granted. The therapist, in conjunction with the patient/client will agree on an appropriate treatment plan, and use purposeful activities to reach their goals. For example, a therapist may teach a person how to dress themselves by alternative methods or using dressing aids following a hip replacement or stroke, or use board games (remedial activities), to improve memory and concentration.

Occupational Therapists also advise on adaptations to the home, from a simple grab rail to bathroom adaptation, stairlift, ramp, kitchen adaptation or ground floor extension. Colleagues from Health, Social Services and Housing Departments work closely together with the client, to plan the most appropriate adaptation to meet the needs of the disabled person. The therapist will also assist with applying for Grants and other sources of funding.

The author of this chapter developed dermatomyositis in 1986, (you may have already read her chapter in this book). She is now, thankfully, fully recovered. As a result of her experience she felt the desire to train as an Occupational Therapist and is now employed by a Social Services Department in Devon. Her principal role is assessing the needs of elderly and disabled people within their own homes. Based on her personal experience and knowledge, this chapter will mainly be focussed on community Occupational Therapy. Hospital Occupational Therapy may perform a different role, but will also be of benefit to those suffering a muscle wasting disease.

How to make contact with an Occupational Therapist

If you are struggling at home, contact your local Social Services Department and make a referral, (request for advice and help). You can do this yourself, or a friend/relative or other professional can do so on your behalf. Most areas of the country will probably have a long waiting list. The demand for input from Social Services is often greater than the resources available; therefore, you will need to check if you are eligible for the provision of a service. Even if the equipment/adaptation/service cannot be provided for you, under the "Chronically Sick and Disabled Persons Act", you are entitled to an *assessment* if you have a permanent and substantial disability. You should, however, be given advice about what/where to purchase services if, following an assessment, Social Services are unable to provide it for you.

The more information you can give about yourself, the easier it will be for the team to make a decision about when you can be seen. For example, if you have a skin condition necessitating regular showering or bathing, or you are incontinent, you may be visited more quickly. If you or your carer is at risk of falling at home and you are unable to meet your basic needs such as getting to the toilet or preparing meals, you may be visited more quickly. An assessment may initially be carried out over the telephone, or a self-assessment form may be sent to you to gather more information. You *may* be asked to pay a contribution to the service using your disability benefits.

How can Occupational Therapy benefit people suffering with a muscle wasting disease?

The role of Occupational Therapy is to help people to help themselves. There are many ways in which you could do this. A muscle wasting disease can be very debilitating, but there may be methods you could adopt to improve your quality of life. Symptoms vary vastly, and some people have periods of flare-ups and remission. The danger is to overdo things when you are feeling well, but this then sets you back and can make you ill. It is not easy to "pace" yourself, especially if you live on your own.

The following information may help you in your home. These are suggestions you might want to consider or pursue further, the author cannot take responsibility for what actions you decide to take and recommends that you ask for an Occupational Therapy assessment if your needs are complex.

Think about your home environment; try to use labour saving equipment, which will help preserve your energy. There are many mobility centres; mail order catalogues and even D.I.Y. stores sell many items of equipment designed for disabled people.

Access – shallower steps with rails may be preferable than a long ramp, unless you need to use a wheelchair. A ramp should be no steeper than 1:12, but if there is room, the shallower the better. There are also other guidelines, so check with your local Housing or Social Services Department. In some cases planning permission may also be required. If your sight is affected, have the edge of steps painted white, or a contrasting colour, which is readily seen. Have good outside lighting.

Mobility– some people with a muscle wasting disease will find walking aids helpful, these range from sticks to frames to wheelchairs. A purpose made trolley is useful for transporting food from the kitchen to the dining room/sitting room and will act as a walking frame as well. (Please note that a standard tea trolley is not usually suitable if you need to lean on it heavily). Grab rails are very useful beside a single step or stair.

Check the height of your chair, if it is difficult to get up from the chair, arrange for it to be raised underneath. This can be a preferable option to raising it with cushions, which will then decrease your back support. There is a good range of electric riser/recline chairs, if your muscles are too weak to be able to push yourself up.

If you are struggling to get in and out of bed, there are a variety of bed rails available. If your difficulties are sitting yourself up in bed, there are pillow and mattress elevators, which can be fitted. Occupational Therapy Technicians will often raise a bed. Profiling beds (beds which go up and down), are also available.

If stairs are difficult, a simple solution could be having a banister rail each side of the stairs. Alternatively, you may need to have a stair lift. There are many stair lift companies and if you have a straight flight of stairs you may be able to have one fitted through a rental scheme. Check whether or not you may be entitled to one through your social services or housing department. You may prefer to sleep downstairs. If this is the case, ensure that you have adequate ventilation for any gas appliances in the room, which may put you at risk. Having a chemical toilet downstairs may reduce the frequency you need to use the stairs, if you do not have a toilet downstairs already.

Toileting – why are toilets so low? Toileting is probably the main activity you will want to continue with dignity and privacy. You may require a grab rail or raised toilet seat to improve the situation. If this is not sufficient, there are devices to help lift you up from the toilet, and models, which will wash and dry you if you cannot manage to keep yourself clean.

Washing/dressing – this is the area in which most people with a disability struggle with. For a person with a muscle wasting disease, a hot bath can be exhausting. However, it may be helpful to aid relaxation and ease pain, plus it may be necessary to use special creams or oils in the bath if you have dermatomyositis. There is a host of bathing equipment on the market, from seats to powered bath lifts, to powered baths and hoists. If you are unable to manage any of these, you may be eligible for a Grant to put in a walk-in shower or have the adaptation carried out by your local Council if you live in a Council property. Referrals can usually only be accepted with the recommendation of an Occupational Therapist.

There is a host of dressing aids, which can readily be borrowed or purchased. Equipment to help you put on your socks or tights, pull up zips, fasten buttons, and dressing sticks are just some of the items. Many suppliers also produce clothing with Velcro fastening or special clothing if you are a wheelchair user. Some disabled people often need the help of home care staff to assist with washing and dressing tasks.

Cooking – extra care needs to be taken when handling hot, heavy pans. Try to re–arrange your kitchen so that the things you use the most are to hand and within easy reach. If possible, have a worktop beside your cooker so you can slide saucepans onto it. Cooking vegetables in a wire basket inside the saucepan is helpful if you have difficulties lifting. This means that you can lift the basket out, drain the vegetables and you can leave the pan to later, when the water has cooled, or wait for someone to help.

Sit down when possible to prepare food or wash up. Look out for the ranges of adapted cutlery and utensils, which will make the task easier and safer. A tabletop cooker or combination microwave oven may be preferable to a low oven thus reducing the risk of falling or dropping hot dishes.

There are now an excellent variety of ready-made meals available in the supermarket if you just cannot cope with cooking yourself. Social Services may deliver meals on wheels if your needs cannot be met in other ways.

Lever taps will be easier to mange if you have a reduced grip. The use of jar openers and electric tin openers will avoid over exertion.

Feeding – if your arms and hands are weak, it can be helpful to rest your forearms on a table whilst you are feeding yourself. Large handled cutlery may be easier to grip. There is also cutlery available with handles set at different angles, and some with straps to go around your fingers. A cup with a straw may be useful or a model with two handles will be easier to use if you have a weak grip. An Occupational Therapist would be able to carry out a feeding and drinking assessment and advise on what equipment best meets your needs. For example, a mobile arm support may help to support your forearm to aid feeding independently.

Domestic activities – if you are fortunate enough to have access to the Internet, most of your shopping can now be bought on-line and delivered to your door. If not, find out who could help or take you to the shops. Shopping can be exhausting, but can be good therapy to do a little if you can. If carrying shopping is a problem, ask at the store if someone can help you, or use a shopping bag on wheels.

Cleaning your home may be a task that you need help with. Also heavier jobs like changing the sheets, doing the laundry, ironing, gardening, and home maintenance, are activities, which you would rather give to someone else. Age Concern, Social Services, Care & Repair, and Anchor Staying Put are examples of organisations, which may be able to give you information about domestic agencies, gardeners and "Handyperson" schemes.

The above is not an exhaustive list, but it is hoped that the information will enable you to think about how you can help yourself and improve your quality of life. Unfortunately there is no known cure (as yet), for muscle wasting diseases, but having the right medication, support, being able to do what you can yourself, and, a positive mind can make all the difference. Just because you have a disability it does not mean you are useless. Try to use your strengths rather than focussing on the negatives.

The role of a Hospital based Therapist

A hospital based Occupational Therapist may be able to make splints for your hands. These will help prevent or correct deformity and help to support your finger and wrist joints when using them. A Physiotherapist may be able to provide ankle or knee supports to wear when mobilising to reduce risk of falls. If you are under the care of a hospital Occupational Therapist you may also be taught fatigue management. This will involve learning how to pace yourself, plan, set priorities and goals and relaxation techniques.

Disability Benefits

Contact your local Benefits Agency (formerly known as the D.S.S.) to ensure you are claiming any Benefits you may be entitled to. Alternatively, there is a Freephone number 0800 88 22 00 to obtain up to date advice and information. Any financial assistance will help you purchase care and services if you want them.

Conclusion

Occupational Therapy seeks to facilitate independence and to enable people to lead purposeful, and more productive lives. Few people appreciate the importance and effectiveness of the Occupational Therapy role. It is hoped that this chapter will have given you an insight into how a person's life can be influenced and changed with the appropriate professional support.

Julie Mallen is a Senior Occupational Therapist with Devon Social Services, UK. She qualified in 1997 following a four year In–Service Course in Occupational Therapy at the University of the West of England, Bristol, Avon, U.K. She has been employed by Social Services for over 12 years.

13

Exercise Treatment in Myositis

by Dr Selwyn Richards BM., BCh (Oxon),
MA (Cantab), MSc., MRCP (UK), DipSportMed (RCSE)
Consultant Rheumatologist, Poole Hospital

This chapter will discuss the general benefits of exercise for the population at large. It then explains the different types of exercise that have been assessed by research in the treatment of myositis. Research studies are then reviewed and conclusions drawn as to which exercises there is best evidence for. Finally, some of the reasons that stop people from getting benefit from exercise are discussed.

'Exercise is good for everyone' – What is the evidence that exercise is good for the population at large and how much exercise do we need to do?

There is general agreement that exercise (for the population at large) 'is a good thing'.

If every adult exercised regularly this would lead to a greater reduction in the number of strokes and heart attacks than if smoking was banned and every smoker was able to stop.

So lack of exercise is the single greatest cause of preventable disease in the western world.

However, it is unclear just how much exercise is enough. In the United Kingdom the government document 'The Health of the Nation' specifically states that it is unclear what exercise is most appropriate even in the highly studied area of heart disease.

In the United States there have been **two** consensus statements that have clearly stated the specific type and duration of exercise recommended for the population as a whole. The **first** was published in 1995;

a thirteen-member panel representing several fields of expertise met to review the evidence. They searched through all available medical evidence and came up with the 'NIH Consensus Statement 1995'. This states:

'All Americans should engage in regular physical activity at a level appropriate to their capacity, needs, and interest. Children and adults alike should set a goal of accumulating at least 30 minutes of moderate-intensity physical activity on most, and preferably, all days of the week. Most Americans have little or no physical activity in their daily lives, and accumulating evidence indicates that physical inactivity is a major risk factor for cardiovascular disease. However, moderate levels of physical activity confer significant health benefits. Even those who currently meet these daily standards may derive additional health and fitness benefits by becoming more physically active or including more vigorous activity. For those with known cardiovascular disease, cardiac rehabilitation programmes that combine physical activity with reduction in other risk factors should be more widely used.'

The **second** American statement on the optimum amount of exercise was given by the American College of Sports Medicine. They suggested that:

'All individuals' health would benefit from an active lifestyle'.

In addition to that, individuals should endeavour to take 30 minutes of exercise, 5 days a week. This is likely to lead to improvement in life expectancy, mood etc. and decreases the risk of heart disease and stroke.

Exercise for people with myositis
Why is myositis bad for your health and not just your muscles?

The bad news about myositis is that sufferers are on average likely to die younger than healthy people of the same age and sex. There is an increase in death rates caused by cancer, heart disease and lung disease as a result of complications of myositis. These sweeping statements however mask a much more complicated picture. There is an increased mortality during the first year after diagnosis and a slower mortality during the following 7 years. Unfavourable prognostic signs in one study have been reported to be failure to induce remission of the muscle disease, high white cell counts in the blood, fever, older age, a shorter disease history and an inability to swallow food.

Traditional 'outdated' advice about exercise in myositis.
There is no agreed consensus as to how much exercise individuals with myositis should do. The conventional wisdom on exercise in myositis has been to encourage rest and gentle joint range of movement. E.A. Awad in his book '*Medical Rehabilitation*' proposed that this is best for the patient in the presence of active disease and a high CPK.

What can we learn from other similar illnesses about exercise?
It has been shown that exercise is beneficial for other inflammatory conditions such as rheumatoid arthritis and lupus. It can lead to less pain, less inflammation and better function. So it is not unreasonable to suggest that exercise may help individuals to become stronger and be able to benefit from the wider effects of exercise on general health.

What types of exercise are there to consider?
There are several different types of exercise that may be beneficial to myositis patients.

Aerobic exercise: also known as cardiovascular fitness. This is most commonly used in exercise referral schemes where general practitioners suggest an exercise scheme through the local leisure centres. Typically this would involve walking or cycling while being able to talk in sentences.

Anaerobic exercise: higher levels of exertion would lead to predominantly anaerobic exercise. Typically one is too breathless to speak in sentences and can only sustain exercise for a few minutes at most.

There are a variety of ways of exercising muscles. Some methods are less intense than others and are less likely to cause muscle damage. For example:

Eccentric contractions involve the muscle trying to contract while being actively lengthened. For example walking down stairs or down hill involves this type of exercise. There are several studies that have shown that such exercise is harmful, leading to tiny tears in the muscle and increased post exercise muscle soreness.

Concentric contractions: this is the opposite to eccentric contractions; and is when the active muscle shortens when contracting. For example lifting a bag up off the floor or walking on the flat or up hill. This tends to limit muscle damage.

Isometric contraction occurs when there is no change in length of the muscle on contraction, as when tensing one's muscles. This may be beneficial initially in increasing muscle strength before any significant additional load can be tolerated. *Isotonic* is when there is no change in resistance. One could have an exercise bike or a rowing machine that however fast you went the effort needed was always the same. It is typically used.

Isokinetic is when there is no change in the speed in which a movement is performed and may be better performed when muscle disease is stable (i.e. not acutely inflamed). So, however hard you try to cycle an exercise bike, the pedals go round at the same speed.

Range of movement exercise i.e. just putting the joints through their pain free movements, without expending any energy is thought to do no harm. This is a good exercise when very active inflammation is present or the muscles are profoundly weak.

Resistive exercise i.e. moving your joints against resistance e.g. getting out of chair is generally a good way of building up strength.

Evidence of the benefits of exercise in myositis
There is published anecdotal evidence of the benefit of isometric exercise. A patient with active stable idiopathic polymyositis received a 4-week supervised right thigh and upper arm isometric strengthening programme. He demonstrated a significant 60% increase in strength without a sustained rise in creatinine phosphokinase (CPK actually fell from 1276 to 834 IU).

Further support came from a study of four patients with polymyositis on high dose prednisolone treated with 12 weeks exercise, alternating 2 weeks resistive exercise (consisting of rolling over, lying to sitting to standing, transfers, walking etc) and passive (range of motion) exercises. Patients were assessed by manual muscle testing (MMT), activities of daily living, maximum strength and CPK. They found that all four showed a mean increase in strength of 60% and that the CPK was elevated only at 2 hours post exercise. There were greater gains in activities of daily living and strength from the resistive exercise.

One issue in polymyositis is whether the amount of exercise that a person can do is limited by other health problems besides their muscle strength. In one study six out of nineteen patients were unable to exercise due to acute myositis (two people), eye problems (one person), a collapsed hip (one person), liver problems (one person), and palpitations caused by thyroid problems (one person). All had normal electrical recordings of the heart and scans of the heart showed their hearts pumped well. Those who were deemed fit to exercise were then exercised to exhaustion. Nine of the eleven stopped their exercise tests limited by muscle fatigue and two were limited by breathlessness. So muscle weakness and fatigue were the commonest attributable causes of exercise limitation. This is important as this is improvable with exercise training.

There have been a couple of slightly larger studies that have looked at the benefits of physiotherapy led aerobic fitness programmes in myositis. In a 6-week study, fourteen patients with dermato- and polymyositis were given exercise training consisting of exercise bicycle and step aerobics. They found this training led to significant improvements in activities of daily living, increased muscle strength and general well being with no flare in disease activity.

Probably the best research study comes from Sweden. It investigated a home exercises programme, which included exercises for strength in the upper and lower limbs, neck and trunk, and for mobility in the upper limbs using stretches. This programme was evaluated in patients with stable, inactive dermato- and polymyositis. Ten patients with reduced muscle function completed the study. The patients exercised for 15 minutes and took a 15-minute walk, 5 days a week, during a 12-week period. After 12 weeks of exercise, there were no signs of increased muscle disease activity as assessed clinically, by CPK values, MRI or muscle biopsy findings. All patients improved regarding muscle function according to a measurement called the "functional index in myositis (FIM)" and also improved in muscle function of the upper and lower limbs, walking distance and general health status.

In summary there have been a small number of studies looking at the effectiveness of exercise in myositis. They have all shown beneficial results, suggesting that **graded fitness exercise is generally safe and beneficial, leading to improvements in strength, well being and fitness.** The limitation of these studies however, is their small size and short duration.

How <u>not</u> to do it

So why is it that so many people who might benefit from exercise don't manage to stick with it? Well there is a recipe for disaster. There are ways of approaching change that set us up for disaster:

Bull buying china

As soon as we know that good can come from change, we go at it full tilt. We go straight to the gym, try and do more than we have done for years, get so exhausted we can hardly get home, can hardly move the next day, even worse the day after that. What do we learn from this experience? Only failure and discouragement.

Think about the past

We are always getting older: change is inevitable. We will never be the person we used to be. If we have been ill, the change is even greater and our expectations of the future must be based on improvement from where we are now, not to where we were once.

Compare self to 'others'

We are all different human beings. No two of us are the same. It's all too easy to see other people succeeding in achieving things that we feel we will never be able to achieve, and be discouraged. Instead we need to set our own goals; what we want and are likely to be able to achieve.

Self talk

Inside our head all the time we are having thoughts. Much of the time these thoughts are running ourselves down. The voice inside our head may be saying:

'I'm lazy.'
'Why make the effort.'
'It's all too difficult.'
'I know this won't work for me.'
'I have tried that before.'
'I have not got the time to spend doing that.'

It is surprising how much of the time we spend putting ourselves down inside our heads. It is important if we are to make changes in our lives that we start to listen to the negative thoughts in our heads. First, we need to recognise that they are there. Then to put some distance from them, counter them with thoughts such as 'I know I tend to run myself down but actually I have been through and achieved much and I don't need to listen to these negative messages'. The next step might be to counteract them with positive messages. 'I know that I can make change and achieve what I want to. I often succeed. I am ready to make a difference in my life'

Put things off
If we don't start a change we will never change. Not starting means not being committed to making a change in our life that might make a difference. So if we want to see change for the better the only time to start is now.

Don't complete the programme
And if we want to succeed we must complete the programme. We must keep to our commitment to a changed way of life. The benefits of exercise only continue as long as we exercise. The consequences of prolonged rest happen quickly. Only one week's rest leads to the loss of 10% of your thigh muscles which will take 3 months to build up again. Unfortunately, most people who start exercise do give up. So to make a change we have to make it a priority.

Don't expose self to fun
We have to enjoy life. Exercise is no different. If it is sociable, if we feel supported, if we reward ourselves for our achievement, we are more likely to persevere and get the most out of it. So if we join a group of similar people, make an effort to talk to people exercising with us, set a target with a reward if we achieve it, we are more likely to succeed.

How to succeed in starting exercise
So the recipe for success when planning to change our life to improve health and so our quality of life is:
- Don't be a bull buying china: take it slowly.
- Think about the present and the future. Plan targets and goals based on what we can do now and what we think we can realistically achieve.

- Don't compare ourselves to 'others'. It's what we want to achieve - not others. We are all individuals.
- Self talk:– we need to recognise the negative things we say to ourselves and replace them with positive 'affirmations'.
- Don't put things off. The future starts today. The future is what we make of it. Certainly events will come along that we did not plan or expect but the more secure we are in the ability to control our own lives and the more influence we see we can have on our own health, the better we may be to handle the unexpected. We need to complete the programme and finally we need to expose ourselves to fun.

Good luck!

Dr Selwyn Richards is a consultant rheumatologist in Poole, Dorset, England. He has a special interest in musculoskeletal pain and fatigue. He completed a three-year research training fellowship funded by the NHS assessing the benefit of exercise prescription in fibromyalgia. He helped set up and run a randomised trial of creatine supplementation and exercise treatment in myositis. In 2001 he was awarded the Young Investigators Award of the British Society of Rheumatology.

14

Exercise Programme

by Helene Alexandersson PhD, PT
Karolinska Institute, Stockholm, Sweden

I have been working as a physiotherapist for 15 years and after see-ing patients with myositis I developed the exercise programme in 1995. The purpose of my thesis, which I did for my PhD, was to eval-uate safety and the effect of different exercise regimes in patients with polymyositis and dermatomyositis and also to develop and evaluate validity and reliability of an assessment tool to measure muscle func-tion and functional limitations in these patients.

Publications relevant to the exercise chapter:

Alexandersson H., Stenstrom C.H., Lundberg I. *Safety of a home exercise programme in patients with polymyositis and dermatomyositis: a pilot study*. Rheumatology 1999: 38:608-11

Alexandersson H., Stenström C.H., Lundberg I. *The safety of a resistive home exercise programme in patients with recent onset active polymyositis or dermatomyositis*. Scan J Rheumatol 2000: 29:295-301.

Alexandersson H., Lundberg I., Stenström C.H. *Development of the myosi-tis activities profile – validity and reliability of a self-administrated ques-tionnaire to assess activity limitations in patients with polymyositis/dermatomyositis*. J Rheumatol 2002: 29:2386-92.

Moderate Exercise Programme for Myositis

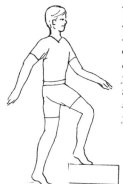

Warming up:
Step up. Use a 20cm high stool. Start with the right leg first during one minute and then change legs. Move your arms as if you were walking. If necessary hold on to something to keep your balance.

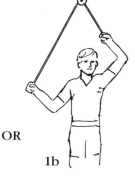

OR

1b

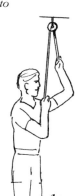

1a. *For mobility in the upper extremities use a pulley apparatus. Push one arm down to help the other up. Work with your elbows forwards-upwards. 10 repetitions per arm.*

OR 1b. *Use the pulley apparatus as above. Work with your elbows sidewards-upwards. 10 repetitions per arm.*

1a

2. *For grip strength hold on to the handles of the pulley apparatus and squeeze them tight with one hand at a time. 10 repetitions per hand.*

3. *For strength in the quadriceps sit on a chair or bed with the thighs supported. If needed put a weight cuff round the ankle. Tense the quadriceps and straighten the knee. Hold for 5 seconds and then relax. 10 repetitions per leg.*

4. *For strength in the shoulder muscles sit on a chair. If needed put weight cuffs around the wrists. Raise one arm at a time above your head as much as you can. 10 repetitions per arm.*

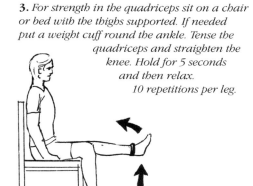

3

4

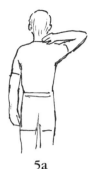

5a. *For mobility and strength in the upper extremities put your hand on your neck. Abduct the arm as much as possible. 10 repetitions per arm.*

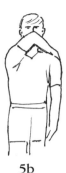

5b. *Hand on the opposite shoulder. Raise the elbow as much as possible. 10 repetitions per arm.*

5c. *Hand on your back. Stretch out as much as you can. 10 repetitions per arm.*

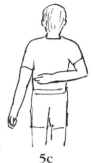

5a   5b   5c

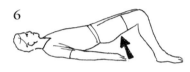

6. *For strength in the lower extremities lay down on the floor or a bed. Bend your knees and push your pelvis up. Hold for 5 seconds and then relax. 10 repetitions.*

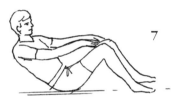

7. *For strength in the trunk muscles lay down with knees bent. Lift your head and tense the trunk muscles and do a sit up. Put your hands up against the knees. If needed, support the neck with one hand. 10 repetitions per arm.*

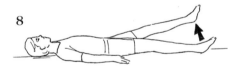

8. *For strength in the hip muscles lay down on your back and lift one leg at a time up about 30cm. In case of low back pain, bend the other knee. 10 repetitions per leg.*

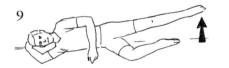

9. *For strength in the hip muscles lay down on one side. Bend one knee and raise the other leg up about 30cm with a straightened knee. 10 repetitions per leg.*

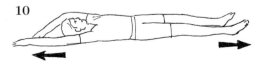

10. *To stretch trunk and shoulder muscles lay down on your back. Put your arms above your head and stretch out one side at a time. Hold for about 20 seconds each side.*

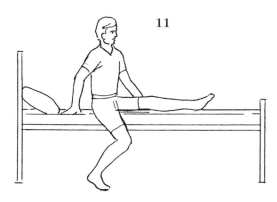

11. *To stretch the hamstrings sit down on a bed. Put one leg up on the bed and put the opposite foot on the floor. Keep your back straight up. Hold for about 20 seconds.*

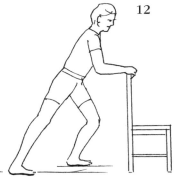

12. *To stretch the calf muscle stand up. Put one foot behind the other and bend the front knee and lean forward against a chair. Keep the heel to the floor all through the exercise. Hold for about 20 seconds. Change sides.*

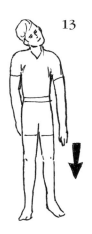

13. *To stretch the neck muscles stand up and lay your ear against your shoulder. Stretch the opposite arm to the floor. Hold for about 20 seconds. Change Sides.*

GOOD LUCK!

With thanks to Helene Alexandersson,
Physical Therapy Department, Rheumatology Unit, Karolinska Hospital, SE-171 76 Stockholm, Sweden.

SECTION FOUR

Understanding the Science

15

The Genetics of Myositis

Hector Chinoy, MRCP, arc Clinical Research Fellow[1,2]

William E. R. Ollier, PhD, FRCPath; Professor of Immunogenetics[2]

Robert G. Cooper, MD, FRCP; Consultant Rheumatologist[1]

1. Introduction

Polymyositis (PM), dermatomyositis (DM) and inclusion body myositis (IBM) are a group of rare systemic diseases forming part of the idiopathic inflammatory myopathies (IIMs), and are characterised by chronic muscle inflammation and weakness. The cause of IIMs are unknown. Although various treatments can all be effective in treating PM/DM, the response varies, and is often disappointing. Patients can occasionally die from their disease, while survivors frequently remain disabled through persisting muscle weakness and/or lung fibrosis. Given the limited effectiveness of the available drugs, new and more potent therapies are clearly needed. However, in the development of new treatments, it is important to first understand the very nature of myositis.

2. Genetic factors

We all possess DNA (deoxyribonuceleic acid), which is a genetic code that our body uses like an instruction manual, in order to make protein with,. A gene is a distinct sequence of DNA, which is transferred from a parent to an offspring, and is responsible for determining the bodily characteristics of offspring, for example eye colour or skin type. DNA is found inside the nucleus of every cell in our bodies, packaged

[1] Rheumatic Diseases Centre, Hope Hospital, Salford
[2] Centre for Integrated Genomic Medical Research, University of Manchester

into tightly formed units called chromosomes. A process called transcription turns DNA into messenger ribonucleic acid (mRNA), which then carries information for the translation into proteins.

We also possess two sets of 23 chromosomes, one from each parent, making a total of 46. The part of a gene from each parent is called an allele. It is when genes become altered, or 'mutated', when problems can arise, and the specific genetic code for a particular function can no longer be translated normally. An example of this is Duchenne muscular dystrophy, an inherited muscle disease, where the gene responsible for making a protein called dystrophin mutates. Dystrophin plays an important structural role in muscle fibre membranes. When the gene mutation occurs, this leads to defective or absent dystrophin protein. A breakdown of muscle tissue then occurs, the result being progressive weakness, and possible death from respiratory muscle failure.

The story is more complicated in autoimmune diseases, such as rheumatoid arthritis, lupus and myositis, as these diseases are thought to be 'polygenic', (i.e. more than one gene appears to be implicated), and 'complex', (i.e. the cause of the disease is not purely genetic). Although genetic factors are implicated in the development of PM/DM, it is likely that genetically predisposed individuals only develop their myositis after environmental exposure to specific triggers. There is an important genetic region, or area, that has been consistently implicated in numerous autoimmune diseases, including rheumatoid arthritis and multiple sclerosis, known as the human leucocyte antigen system, or HLA, (also called the major histocompatibility complex (MHC)), which is found on chromosome 6. Three distinct regions have been identified; classes I, II and III. HLA class I incorporates HLA-A, -B and -C genes, class II incorporates HLA-DQ and -DR genes, and class III includes tumour necrosis factor (TNF) genes. The current evidence to suggest a genetic basis for IIMs is now summarised.

2.1 Familial Aggregation

Most of the evidence for familial aggregation comes from 35 case descriptions in the literature. The first description of familial disease was by Wedgwood in 1953, who described the onset of juvenile DM in twins within one year of each other. Other families have since been described, where two or more members have an IIM.

One investigation of multicase families with myositis suggested that clinical, antibody and genetic features differ between familial and non-familial (patients without a myositis relative i.e. the vast majority of myositis patients) disease (1). The theory is that if familial patients should share genetic risk factors with each other, and perhaps possess greater genetic risk of disease than non-familial patients with the disease 'running in the family'. Dr Fred Miller's group investigated 36 patients with familial PM, DM or IBM, who were identified from 16 unrelated families, where at least 2 family members possessed myositis (1). These familial IIM cases were compared with 181 patients with non-familial myositis. Myositis antibodies were detected more frequently in non-familial myositis. The genetic allele HLA-DRB1*0301* has an odds ratio (OR) of 9.5 in non-familial myositis, i.e. they are 9.5 times more likely than the general population to develop myositis. Likewise, a non-familial individual with DQA1*0501 has an OR of 4.9, i.e. they are 4.9 times more likely than the general population to develop myositis. In contrast, only the allele DRB1*0301 was a risk factor in familial disease, with an OR of 5.5. The possession of 2 identical alleles, which is called homozygosity, in the DQA region, appeared to be a unique risk factor for familial disease. The familial and non-familial groups of patients share many features, but the few differences found may suggest the importance of unidentified environmental and genetic factors in the cause of sporadic myositis.

A further study looked at the frequency of different autoimmune diseases amongst first degree relatives with non-familial myositis (2). The prevalence of autoimmune diseases (e.g. autoimmune thyroid disease, diabetes, rheumatoid arthritis) was about five times higher in first-degree relatives of patients with myositis, than in relatives of non-myositis patients. The spectrum of different autoimmune diseases was of similar distribution to that seen in the general population.

2.2 Candidate Gene Studies

The best current evidence for a genetic basis in causing myositis comes from candidate gene studies, comparing myositis populations to matched controls. A candidate gene is one which is suspected of

*HLA-DRB1*0301 is a particular allele found in the HLA region on chromosome 6.

having a specific role in causing disease. These studies confirm the MHC region to have the strongest association with myositis, similar to findings in other autoimmune diseases. The first of these studies looked at HLA class I. More recent studies using molecular polymerase chain reaction (PCR) based techniques have demonstrated that genes in HLA class II, DRB1*0301 and DQA1*0501 are important risk factors for myositis in Caucasian adults and children.

Myositis HLA associations seen in Caucasians are not found in other ethnic populations. For example, no HLA associations have been found in Mexican-American, Korean and Hispanic myositis populations. This emphasises the importance of performing genetic studies in single ethnic groups. Rider et al compared HLA-DR and DQ in a white American and Korean population (3). The expected associations with HLA-DRB1*0301 and DQA*0501 were found in the white population, but no association was found in the Korean population, even though both sets of patients had similar sets of clinical characteristics and autoantibody profiles.

2.3 UK AOMIC Study

The majority of previous IIM candidate gene studies have analysed adult and juvenile PM/DM patient results together, and some studies have even included results from IBM patients. Such grouping, which reflects the rarity of these diseases, is undertaken to increase study sample sizes and gain power during statistical comparisons of IIM patients with control subjects. Given the differences (i.e. of clinical, antibody and pathological features) between IIM sub-types, a more logical approach would be to compare and contrast, rather than group, these diseases during genetic comparisons. To get over the sample size problems, and address the question of whether PM and DM are genetically the same with respect to HLA class II, we recently coordinated a UK nationwide collaborative study of 59 physicians, which has been known as the UK 'Adult Onset Myositis Immunogenetic Collaboration' (AOMIC). This has recruited 110 PM and 98 DM UK Caucasian patients since 2000. These patients' HLA-DRB1 data has been compared with those of 537 ethnically matched controls. The results confirmed that HLA-DRB1*03 was a risk factor for PM with an OR of 4.0 *(Table 1)*.

Table 1: Immunogenetic risk factors in UK AOMIC cohort

	Controls n=537	Polymyositis n=110		Dermatomyositis n=98	
HLA	n(%)	n(%)	probability	n(%)	probability
DRB1*03	151 (28.1)	67 (60.9)	3×10^{-11}	43 (43.9)	0.002
DRB1*07	129 (24.0)	9 (8.2)	1×10^{-04}	36 (36.7)	0.008

However, there was also a significant protective effect of HLA-DRB1*07 in PM versus controls with an OR of 0.3. The results for DM patients were different, as the association with HLA-DRB1*03 was considerably weaker than for PM, with an OR of 2.0 and, by contrast with PM, DRB1*07 represented a risk factor versus controls, OR 1.8. These results suggest that in a UK Caucasian population, HLA-DRB1 plays a role in governing PM/DM disease susceptibility, through association with DRB1*03, and may also govern the expression of myositis disease type, through association with DRB1*07. These are only preliminary results and further associations are currently being investigated.

2.4 HLA Associations with Myositis Autoantibodies

Groups of myositis specific antibodies (MSAs) may define specific subsets of patients according to clinical status, prognosis and response to treatment. Certain HLA class II alleles may also act as risk factors in the development of these antibodies. Arnett et al examined antibody subsets in four differing ethnic groups with myositis (4). The association of HLA class II in Caucasian patients appeared to be stronger in patients positive for anti-Jo-1 antibody or other MSAs. HLA-DQA1 showed stronger associations along ethnic lines, and it was felt therefore that this allele was associated with the expression of certain MSAs.

2.5 Other Genetic Associations

Tumour necrosis factor alpha (TNFα) is a pro-inflammatory cytokine[†], and has an important role in regulation of the overall immune

[†]Cytokine: A soluble factor carrying information and signals locally between cells

response to infection. The TNFα-308A allele is associated with an increase in TNFα synthesis, which may cause increased susceptibility to various infections and a higher relapse rate of non-Hodgkin's lymphoma. In a study of juvenile DM children (JDM), the TNFα-308A allele was demonstrated in 18/36 patients, and was associated with a long disease course (73% with long course vs 13% with short disease course), with an OR of 17.3 and pathological calcifications (5). An association of this gene has also been found in adult patients.

Muscle fibres in biopsies from IIM patient, and in cultured muscle cells, express HLA-G, a non-classical MHC class I molecule. HLA-G is undetectable in normal muscle, but is found in muscle fibres, inflammatory cells and capillaries in PM, DM and IBM. HLA-G is thought to play an important role in immune tolerance, and more specifically, may help prevent maternal immune cells from attacking the foetus in pregnancy. HLA-G1 and -G5 have been demonstrated as powerful inhibitors of the immune responses (6), and in the future these molecules could form the basis of a muscle cell protective agent for reducing IIM cell-mediated injury.

2.6 Microchimerism

Microchimerism refers to the presence of two genetically distinct and separately derived populations of cells, one population being at a low concentration, in the same individual. Microchimerism may be due to transfer of cells between mother and foetus or between two twins. Maternal microchimeric cells (i.e. maternal cells persisting in offspring) have been found in the peripheral blood and muscle lesions of juvenile IIM patients. In a recent study of HLA and maternal microchimerism in JDM (7), maternal chimeric cells were identified in 60/72 (83%) of JDM patients, versus 5/29 (17%) of healthy male controls, OR 24. All healthy siblings with microchimerism were either HLA-DQA1*0501 positive, or had non-inherited (maternal) DQA1*0501 cells present. The risk for JDM and other autoimmune diseases may therefore be determined by the HLA genotype of the mother, providing a 'second hit' to trigger disease in genetically susceptible individuals. The inherited HLA genotype may therefore contribute to loss of immune self-tolerance, activation of chimeric cells, and starting the disease process and inflammation.

The finding of loss of tolerance is in contrast to other situations where chimerism may be beneficial, such as pregnancy or organ transplantation. An interesting analogy of microchimerism is that of chronic graft-versus-host disease (GVHD), a complication of bone marrow transplants where donor cells in the bone marrow graft attack the host's tissues. Patients undergoing haematopoietic stem cell transplantation (a form of bone marrow transplantation) over a 30-year period have been retrospectively reviewed (8). Of the 1859 patients who developed GVHD, 12 also developed a myositis syndrome (GVHD-PM), resembling idiopathic PM in many clinical and laboratory aspects. Not one of the stem cell transplant patients without GVHD developed myositis. The cases of GVHD-PM, and their resemblance to IIM, suggest a common underlying pathogenesis in both conditions, with microchimeric cells in IIM forming the role of donor cells, and this bolsters the hypothesis that myositis represents an allo-immune mediated disease.

3. 'Elemental Disorders'

It was previously thought that genetically predisposed individuals only develop their autoimmune diseases after certain interactions with environmental triggers, so is there any recent evidence to support this? Previous work has suggested that where you live and at what latitude may influence the type of myositis that you get, i.e. DM rather than PM. The findings of a more recent paper by Dr Fred Miller's team (9) are of great interest. In studying 919 IIM patients in 15 global locations for 13 different climatic variables, surface ultraviolet (UV) light intensity (amount of sunlight exposure) proved the strongest contributor to the relative proportion of DM compared to PM, and to the relative proportion of a particular antibody subset (anti-Mi-2 antibodies). So it appears that the greater an individual's exposure to sunlight, the greater the likelihood that should the individual develop myositis, it would be anti-Mi-2 positive DM in type. These remarkable results suggest that an environmental factor may be capable of modulating the expression of both the clinical and immunological features of the resulting myositis. The authors speculate that sunlight achieves this by playing a role in the development of Mi-2 antibodies (and therefore DM as well), via UV affected cells in the immune system. The presence of anti-Mi-2 antibodies in DM patients are very strongly associated with the allele HLA-DRB1*0701. Dr Miller describes the concept of 'elemental disorders', where autoimmune diseases are the result of interactions between genetic and elemental environmental risk factors to produce unique sign-symptom complexes.

4. Inclusion body myositis

As IBM usually presents with distal (extremities), rather than proximal (shoulder/pelvis), muscle weakness, and thus mimicking nerve damage, it is more commonly seen by neurologists than rheumatologists (at least in the UK). However, due to presence of inflammation in muscle biopsies, IBM is considered one of the IIMs. Several HLA alleles are already known to be risk factors for sporadic IBM. There are currently no clinical or biochemical parameters that predict the outcome of IBM or response to treatment, and HLA typing may in the future help subgroup IBM patients and predict such parameters.

Sporadic IBM muscle biopsies possess structural abnormalities similar to those in brain tissue from Alzheimer's disease patients, including deposition of an abnormal protein called amyloid. A novel gene transfer technique has been used to transfer amyloid into muscle fibres, which caused abnormalities similar to those found in IBM, suggesting a key role of this protein. The same gene was transferred into muscle fibres from a patient with known sporadic IBM and associated cardiac amyloid disease, who already had a further amyloid genetic mutation (transthyretin [TTR]). The resulting overexpression of the gene amplified the abnormalities found in this patient's cultured muscle fibres, which were over and above those seen in the normal muscle experiments. The TTR mutation could either be a genetic risk factor, or perpetuate the existing IBM.

5. Alternative and future approaches

An approach using new available technologies would make use of gene expression microarray profiling. This method allows thousands of genes to be evaluated simultaneously, representing a major genomic advance in surveying tissues for alteration in gene expression. The production of mRNA from a gene reflects the use of that gene, and the potential of being translated into protein. Measurement of the steady state of mRNA provides an indication of which genes are up- or down-regulated. The technology has already yielded a number of studies in myositis patients. This approach may allow hypotheses and models to be generated, leading to elucidation of disease mechanisms. For example, as a result of expression profiling, juvenile DM is thought to incorporate a number of models involving interruption of the blood supply, action against a possible virus, and a process of muscle fibre degeneration. In the future, improved techniques and reduced costs may allow powerful high density techniques to scan the whole human genome (i.e. all of the DNA that an individual possesses) using a single 'gene-chip' for each patient. Gene-chips have already been developed which allow the simultaneously testing of 100,000 genes. Ideally a myositis study would be carried out prospectively and in one centre, so that assessment tools could carefully follow response to treatment and clinical course. This would prove extremely difficult on a practical basis, due to the rarity of myositis, and require several years of patient recruitment in order to gain sufficient numbers. This rarity has prevented the use of more traditional genetic methods, which have been extensively used in the investigation of other rheumatic diseases.

6. Conclusions

The genetic work being undertaken around the world demonstrates the advantages, and indeed necessity, of undertaking national/international genetic collaborations. The results of these larger studies illustrate the importance during genetic testing of treating IIM subtypes as discrete, rather than grouped, diagnoses. Due to the rarity of IIMs, only further collaboration is likely to elucidate the complex interactions between genetic and environmental factors. The mechanistic research will hopefully increase our understanding of the underlying pathogenesis of the IIMs. A basic science approach led to the elucidation of the key role of TNFα in rheumatoid arthritis, and the subsequent development of anti-TNFα therapy. By analogy, ongoing collaborative genetic work may help identify key hierarchical molecules implicated in IIM pathology.

7. Reference list

(1) Rider LG, Gurley RC, Pandey JP, Garcia dlT, I, Kalovidouris AE, O'Hanlon TP *et al*. *Clinical, serologic, and immunogenetic features of familial idiopathic inflammatory myopathy*. Arthritis Rheum 1998; 41(4):710-719.

(2) Ginn LR, Lin JP, Plotz PH, Bale SJ, Wilder RL, Mbauya A *et al*. *Familial autoimmunity in pedigrees of idiopathic inflammatory myopathy patients suggests common genetic risk factors for many autoimmune diseases*. Arthritis Rheum 1998; 41(3):400-405.

(3) Rider LG, Shamim E, Okada S, Pandey JP, Targoff IN, O'Hanlon TP *et al*. *Genetic risk and protective factors for idiopathic inflammatory myopathy in Koreans and American whites: a tale of two loci*. Arthritis Rheum 1999; 42(6):1285-1290.

(4) Arnett FC, Targoff IN, Mimori T, Goldstein R, Warner NB, Reveille JD. *Interrelationship of major histocompatibility complex class II alleles and autoantibodies in four ethnic groups with various forms of myositis*. Arthritis Rheum 1996; 39(9):1507-1518.

(5) Pachman LM, Liotta-Davis MR, Hong DK, Kinsella TR, Mendez EP, Kinder JM *et al*. *TNFalpha-308A allele in juvenile dermatomyositis: association with increased production of tumor necrosis factor alpha, disease duration, and pathologic calcifications*. Arthritis Rheum 2000; 43(10):2368-2377.

(6) Wiendl H, Mitsdoerffer M, Hofmeister V, Wischhusen J, Weiss EH, Dichgans J *et al*. *The non-classical MHC molecule HLA-G protects human muscle cells from immune-mediated lysis: implications for myoblast transplantation and gene therapy*. Brain 2003; 126(Pt 1):176-185.

(7) Lambert NC, Evans PC, Hashizumi TL, Maloney S, Gooley T, Furst DE *et al*. *Cutting edge: persistent fetal microchimerism in T lymphocytes is associated with HLA-DQA1*0501: implications in autoimmunity*. J Immunol 2000; 164(11):5545-5548.

(8) Stevens AM, Sullivan KM, Nelson JL. *Polymyositis as a manifestation of chronic graft-versus-host disease*. Rheumatology 2003; 42(1):34-39.

(9) Okada S, Weatherhead E, Targoff IN, Wesley R, Miller FW. Global surface ultraviolet radiation intensity may modulate the clinical and immunologic expression of autoimmune muscle disease. Arthritis Rheum 2003; 48(8):2285-2293.

16

Diagnosing Myositis – A Laboratory Perspective

Yannoulla Wilson, CSci, FIBMS, Head BMS - Clinical Immunology, NWLH Trust

Dr C. Bernard Colaço

Introduction

The human body has developed systems to protect it *(self)* from the invasion of foreign environmental organisms, which include bacteria, viruses, parasites and fungi *(pathogens)*. These pathogens would normally be eliminated by our natural immune defences, targeting foreign bits of the organism *(antigens)*. This immune system mediated process produces antibodies. These are specific proteins which bind a particular antigen and assist in its destruction.

Autoimmunity

The immune system can, however, misfire and may target its own body parts, such as cells, tissues and even large organs which are mistakenly seen as foreign substances. These autoantibodies (from the Greek *"auto"* meaning *self*) are potentially damaging if other systems which come into action are also activated, such as complement proteins and certain white blood cells. Autoantibodies made in lymph glands and similar tissues may travel in the blood stream and accumulate in target tissues, initiating destruction of those tissues. Other factors influencing this process include genetic propensity, hormone status and triggers such as previous viral infections.

In myositis, immune active cells may be directly involved in causing damage (see chapter 2 – Jo Cambridge) but the study of autoantibodies can be helpful in recognising the type of process as immune mediated and help to classify the patient at an early stage. Despite these tests, it remains a complex clinical picture which requires blood testing for muscle damage (creatine kinase levels) and non-specific inflammation (ESR, CRP). Blood testing for disease-specific autoantibody markers, as well as muscle biopsy and electromyography (EMG) are also needed, and help to clinch the diagnosis.

Muscle Biopsy

Muscle biopsies can be taken quite simply under local anaesthetic with a needle punch technique, but it is often preferable to take an 'open' surgical biopsy which is slightly larger and allows the sample to be handled better by the laboratory for a wider range of testing. Patients may be required to have an MRI scan so the most active muscle can be selected, because muscle damage can be patchy and the small sample may miss the involved tissue.

Diagnostic criteria

In the laboratory, the histopathologist will look at the gross structure of muscle fibres, the blood vessels supplying it and any sign of abnormal immune cells infiltrating the muscle tissue. An early sign of muscle necrosis is the loss of normal striations (cross-markings) and migration of the nucleus from the periphery into the centre of the cells (*Figure 1*). Other tests include staining for levels of specific muscle enzymes and very high powered microscopy with an electron microscope. These may be diagnostic, for instance in inclusion body myositis (IBM) but also help to exclude muscular-dystrophies, which sometimes mimic inflammatory myositis. In *Figure 2*, you will see the typical inclusion bodies in vacuoles of IBM.

Figure 1
Normal muscle showing striations. One of the earliest signs of myofibre necrosis is the loss of these striations.

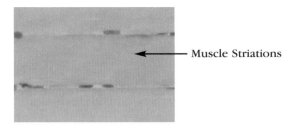

Muscle Striations

Figure 2
IBM Muscle Biopsy

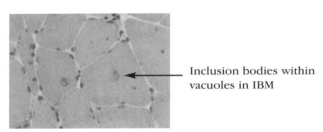

Inclusion bodies within
vacuoles in IBM

Polymyositis/Dermatomyositis)

There can be a spectrum of pathology between PM and DM but necrosis (dying and dead cells) and atrophy, and abnormal migration of the cell nucleus can be common to both. Further detailed tests will show evidence of blood vessel involvement (vasculitis) more commonly in DM, and the ratio of infiltrating T-cells may either be predominantly CD8 in PM, towards CD4 in DM, but never exclusively so. In *Figure 3*, the fluorescence highlights a complex of antibodies and complement proteins surrounding a blood vessel and causing muscle damage (Membrane Attack Complex).

Figure 3
Identification of Membrane Attack Complex (MAC) in the vessel of a DM muscle biopsy

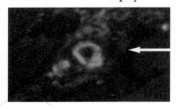

Membrane Attack
Complex

Autoantibodies in Myositis

It is worth noting that inflammatory myositis and a closely related condition, (SLE) may both lead to specific multi-organ damage (skin, lung and muscles). However the antibodies identified are directed at very specific proteins and bits of the genetic code structure which are found in the nucleus and cytoplasm of most cells in the body, i.e. these are 'non-organ' specific autoantibodies. The reader may be helped by *Diagram 1*, 'The Cell', to recognise the positive tests shown later, which do depend on certain laboratory techniques of highlighting or exaggerating the antigen in the test tissue so as not to miss weak positive blood samples which are none-the-less very specific for these abnormalities. In *Figure 4*, a,b,c, we recognise broad patterns of different antibody actions which lead the laboratory scientist to do further testing for more specific ELISAs and other techniques to identify levels of highly specific binding to unique intra-cellular particles. The anti-nuclear antibody (ANA) has been recognised since the 1950s, and revolutionised the clinico-pathological diagnosis of the spectrum of immune-mediated disorders.

Diagram 1
The Cell

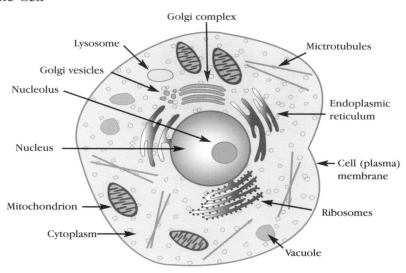

The ANA Immunofluorescence Procedure

The technique of immunofluorescence which gives us these illustrative pictures (*Figures 3-6*) is based on a simple principle of testing the patient's blood serum on a tissue on a laboratory slide. If there is binding of patient's autoantibody, i.e. positive test, it is detected by another layer of fluorescent agent which makes it visible under the microscope (*Diagram 2*).

Diagram 2

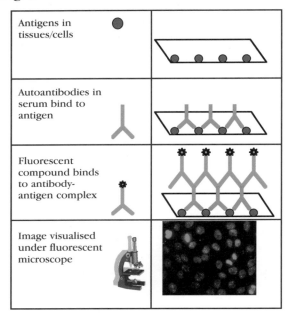

I have included illustrative pictures in *Figure 5*, to show the specificity of binding for nuclear proteins at different stages of a cell cycle.

Historically, the big advance in the 1980s was recognising the Jo-1 antigen (*Figure 6*) belonged to a family of specific enzymes used in the cell to charge part of the genetic coding process of protein production., e.g histdyl-tRNA synthetase, now noted in 15-25% in adult patients with PM, and often linked to inflammatory lung disease and joint pain. For those of you interested in collecting stamps, you will enjoy *Table 1*, which lists some of the other interesting antigens which are diagnostically helpful, and if you are still strong enough for *Table 2*, you will appreciate the increasing complexity in autoimmune testing in myositis.

Figure 4

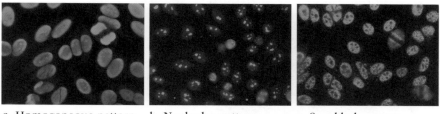

a. Homogeneous pattern   b. Nucleolar pattern   c. Speckled pattern

Figure 5

Anti Nuclear Antibody patterns exposed during the different stages of the cell cycle

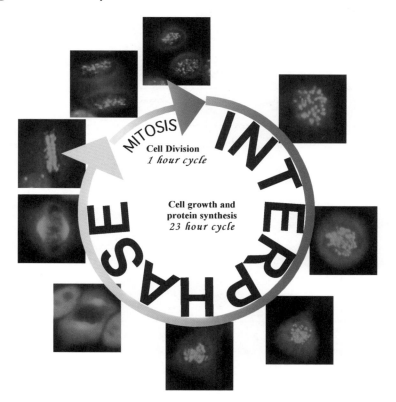

Figure 6
Typical immunofluorescent pattern of anti-Jo-1 antibody

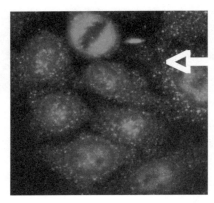

◁— Cytoplasmic Staining

Table 1
Myositis-Associated Autoantibodies

Autoantibody	Immunofluorescence pattern	Antigen	Clinical Associations	Clinical incidence	Specificity
Ku	Nuclear Homogeneous	2 proteins: 60-70 kD 80-86 kD	• Japanese • PM/Scleroderma overlap • Raynaud's • Lung disease	30%	99%
U1nRNP	Nuclear Speckled	22, 33, 70 kD proteins	• PM/DM • CTD overlap syndrome	4-17%	
PM/Scl	Nucleolar & Nuclear Homogeneous	PM/Scl-75 PM/Scl-100	• PM • PM/Scleroderma overlap syndrome	8% 50%	
SSA/Ro	Nuclear & Cytoplasmic Speckled	52, 60 kD proteins	• PM/DM • SLE/Sjogren's overlap syndrome	5-10% 30-50%	

Table 2
Myositis-Specific Autoantibodies

Autoantibody	Immunofluorescence pattern	Antigen	Clinical Associations	Clinical incidence	Specificity
Jo-1	Cytoplasmic Speckled	Histidyl-tRNA synthetase	• PM • Lung disease • Arthralgia • 'Mechanic's hands' syndrome • Responsive to steroids	15-25%	>95%
PL-7	Cytoplasmic Speckled	Threonyl-tRNA synthetase	• PM/DM • Lung disease	3-5%	
PL-12	Dense Cytoplasmic Speckled	Alanyl-tRNA synthetase-	• PM/DM • Lung disease	2-3%	
EJ	Cytoplasmic	Glycyl-tRNA synthetase	• PM • DM	2% 2%	80%
OJ	? Probably cytoplasmic	Isoleucyl tRNA synthetase	• PM/DM	<2%	
SRP	Dense Cytoplasmic Speckled + Nucleolus	Signal Recognition Particles 54kD Protein	• PM • Acute severe onset • Cardiac involvement • Unresponsive to steroids • Black females	4%	93%
Mi-2	Nuclear speckled	235-240 kD	• DM • Nailfold lesions • Respond to steroids	10-20%	

(Grey boxes: Autoantibody profiles still undergoing research or identified in specialist centres.)

I started my training in Histopathology at Central Middlesex Hospital in 1975 and gained Fellowship of the Institute of Biomedical Sciences in 1981. I gained a particular interest in autoimmune disease whilst working there and set up the autoimmune laboratory service in 1979. I was a founder member of the Rheumatology Self-Help group with Dr Colaço at CMH and remain an active participant. After the merger between Central Middlesex and Northwick Park hospitals, I was transferred to the Northwick Park site in December 2002 where I was responsible for setting up and running the full immunology service for the whole Trust. I am currently doing the Diploma of Expert Practice in Immunology and hope to gain expert status by April 2006.

Yannoulla Wilson

17

Myositis in Children

by Susan Maillard, Specialist in Paediatric Rheumatology

and Lucy R Wedderburn, Reader and Consultant in Paediatric Rheumatology

Rheumatology Unit, Great Ormond Street Hospital for Children and Institute of Child Health, UCL, 30 Guilford Street, London WC1N 1EH

Types of myositis in children

Myositis is rare in children, and it affects about 3 children per million each year. In the UK this means that there are between 40 and 50 new cases of myositis in children in each year. It is more common in girls than boys and often starts between the ages of 4 and 9 years. Within the group of children who do get myositis, one type of the illness, called juvenile dermatomyositis, is by far the most common. Polymyositis and inclusion body myositis are both extremely rare in children. Therefore this chapter will focus mostly on juvenile dermatomyositis, which is also known as JDM. Partly because it is so rare, JDM may be mistaken for other illnesses at the start. This is discussed more below. In this chapter we will describe how the illness may start, how it is different from myositis in adults, and then the tests that a child may need to have done if JDM is suspected, and how modern treatments and management can improve the lives of children with myositis.

How the condition can start : the common and the more rare symptoms

The most common symptoms that often happen at the start of JDM are a rash and gradually increasing weakness of the muscles. However in many children these two do not start at exactly the same time, so that the rash may come on before the weakness or vice versa. The rash can be most easily recognised when it is typically on the knuckles backs of hands or knees, but other rashes almost anywhere on the body can occur. Unfortunately the rash can easily be mistaken for some other skin problem such as psoriasis and this can lead to a delay in the child being seen by a specialist. In addition to the typical rash the skin can be affected in other ways such as with areas of break down (ulceration) of the skin or a thickening under the skin that is called calcinosis.

In children, weakness can be mistaken for tiredness or even lack of will. Therefore careful testing of muscle strength is needed, by trained staff, to pick up early weakness as otherwise this can also be missed. As well as the rash and weakness, children with JDM are often very tired, may have mood changes and or irritability. Other parts of the body can also be affected, such as the gut or throat, which can lead to problems such as difficulty in swallowing or a change in the voice.

Children with JDM can also have other symptoms and often these do not all start at the same time. A child with JDM can have fevers, can get painful swollen joints, (a type of arthritis) and can get stomach pains. In fact JDM can affect many other organs in the body including lungs, heart or brain but these complications are more rare than the typical rash and weakness. Since the different aspects of JDM can come on at different times, they are not always recognised for being part of the illness right away. As well as this, it is quite common for children with myositis to have other features that are more typical of another condition, such as for example scleroderma or an illness called lupus. These children, who are sometimes said to have 'overlap' conditions, may have an illness which then gradually changes as they get older. It is not yet understood why these 'overlap' conditions seem to be more common in children than adults with DM. Another difference between adults and children with DM is that in children with DM there is no association with cancer.

Tests a child might have to help make the diagnosis of myositis
Once JDM is suspected it is important that a child is seen by a specialist who has experience in this field. More and more, in the UK this means that the child will be seen by a team known as Paediatric

Rheumatologists, but very often the child is first seen by a children's doctor (a Paediatrician) who then makes a referral to the specialist. In order to help confirm the diagnosis the team will need to examine the child carefully, as well as do blood tests, and possibly a special scan of the muscles, called an MRI, or take a small piece of muscle tissue (known as a biopsy). In younger children, the scans are generally done while the child is asleep under a general anaesthetic and muscle biopsy is always under an anaesthetic. In a few hospitals doctors may do an electrical test known as an EMG, but this is used less in children than in adults. Since myositis is rare in children, experts in the field are working together from around the world to try to agree upon ways to make the diagnosis and also ways to measure how mild or severe the condition is for any one child. This is done using agreed measurements and methods such as the CMAS (Childhood Myositis Assessment Score) which involves a series of defined tasks like sit ups or raising the head off the bed for a time. In combination with testing of the strength of the muscles directly, which is called manual muscle testing, to grade the strength of specific muscles, these tests mean that the weakness can be measured in an accurate way. Having internationally agreed ways to define and measure myositis in children is very important to allow good research to be done into how best to look after and treat these children. You can find further information about some of these international efforts on the website of the Paediatric Rheumatology International Trials Organisation (also called PRINTO): *www. printo.it/pediatric–rheumatology/*

How childhood myositis is treated

One of the most important aspects of the care of children with myositis is that it is now agreed by most professionals working in this area that these children should be looked after in specialist centres where a team of experts are available. The team is likely to include doctors, specialist physiotherapists, nurses, and also for some children, speech therapists, occupational therapists and psychologists. This list reflects the many possible aspects of JDM. However in order to access these specialist teams, it has to be recognised for any individual child that he or she may have JDM and they need to be referred for an opinion. Sometimes this still takes a long time, in part since GP's or other health professionals may not have seen a case before. For this reason experts interested in the field came together in 2000 to form a network of those working in the area, know as the UK juvenile dermatomyositis research Group (JDRG). A national collection of information about children with myositis now exists, that is called the UK and Ireland UK National Registry and Repository for JDM, and this has greatly increased the sharing of information across the UK for those involved in caring for children with JDM.

Once a child has had myositis confirmed, treatments are available. Most children are given steroids, either into a drip and or as tablets, but nowadays it is always the aim to keep the time of steroid treatment as short as possible. The addition of other medicines such as one called methotrexate, usually given as a weekly injection, can much reduce the amount of steroids needed. In severe cases other medicines such as cyclophosphamide or ciclosporin, are considered. Some of these medicines may require a child to stay in hospital for treatment. However the goals of treatment are to help a child to return to school and full active life as rapidly as possible.

It is now understood that it is important to treat the condition as quickly and as fully as possible with the aim of regaining muscle power and function. In parallel with medical treatment, exercise is an integral part of the management of these children, as discussed below.

Physiotherapy for Juvenile Dermatomyositis.

JDM causes problems with muscles that do not work with the same strength as before and joints that do not move fully and often the child can become very tired and moody very quickly. Exercise was previously thought to be harmful to children with active JDM; however this was not supported by any medical evidence and now the evidence positively encourages early interventions with exercises. In fact it is now understood that many children with JDM, even if they get very weak when the condition starts, can regain full strength if they have adequate physiotherapy and exercise.

During the early stages of the disease, when it is quite active, the child may be moderately or severely weak. The exercises at this time should be aimed towards keeping all joints moving fully and encouraging each child to move by themselves as much and as safely possible. As the medicines start to work and the child becomes stronger; measured by an increase in the CMAS (see above), the exercises will take on a different focus: In the recovery phase, as the child is increasing his or her strength, the exercise will encourage this process of recovery and the programme will be aimed at increasing specific muscle strength and fitness. These exercises will work using the evidence for muscle training for children, and will be based on a high repetition programme (to improve stamina of each muscle) and graduated weights/resistance (to improve the strength of each muscle). Full range of movement of each joint will also be maintained at this phase.

Evidence has shown that children with JDM, even though the active disease is well controlled, still continue to have difficulties related to loss of general fitness and endurance and some specific muscle wasting may remain. Therefore it is important for each child to have an exercise programme that works on the specific muscles that are weak and that they are encouraged to join in sporting activities. The specific programme should be a high repetition and low weights programme and the sporting activities ideally need to be low impact and high aerobic sports such as swimming and cycling, though when the child has regained full strength and fitness all sports may be possible.

The evidence base for exercise therapy in children.
All the evidence for training children to increase strength and fitness indicates that they do most effectively with a programme that incorporates high repetitions (i.e. how many times you do each exercise and the more repetitions completed the greater the stamina gained, often a minimum of 15 and a maximum of 30 is indicated). To improve strength, resistance should be added and this is often done with the use of weights. Initially a 0.5kg weight can be added and then increased regularly (either 1x week or 1x fortnight) by 0.5kg to a maximum of 2.5kg (though the age and size of the child needs to be considered when the maximum is achieved).

Other considerations in treatment and management
Children with JDM can have difficulties walking, either because they are too weak or because they get tired easily. It is therefore extremely important that they have good supportive footwear to support their

feet and ankles. Ankle lace–up boots / trainers are the most appropriate and will provide both comfort and support. During the acute phase of the disease there may be many things that a child with JDM can no longer do for themselves and therefore they may require the help of an occupational therapist in order to make suggestions of different ways of completing tasks as well as temporarily lending equipment in order to make life as easy as possible.

In conclusion, the recognition and treatment of JDM has improved considerably in the last 10 years and there are an increasing number of specialist teams around the country who have experience of treating children with myositis. However there is still some distance to go. We still do not know what causes JDM and work is actively carrying on to understand this as well as to find ways of predicting which children will suffer from the more severe complications. Although children with JDM can be initially very severely limited in their independent activities during the active phase, with the correct medical and physiotherapeutic treatments, most children will regain full and independent lives with minimal difficulties remaining. This is the goal of early and active treatment.

18

Inclusion Body Myositis

by Dr John F. McCarthy Mb BCh BAO (NUI), MRCPI
Specialist Registrar in Rheumatology & General
Medicine London Deanery (1999)
and Dr C. Bernard Colaço BSc (Hons) MBChB FRCP

O f all the diseases classified under the title 'Idiopathic Inflam–matory Myositis' (Table 1) Inclusion Body Myositis (IBM) remains at once the most intriguing and frustrating. Presentation may be delayed, diagnosis can be difficult and ultimately treatment or perhaps, more correctly, management can be disappointing.

Table 1

Idiopathic Inflammatory Myositis
• Primary Idiopathic Polymyositis
• Primary Idiopathic Dermatomyositis
• Polymyositis/Dermatomyositis associated with malignancy
• Polymyositis/Dermatomyositis associated with autoimmune disease
• Inclusion Body Myositis

While IBM does share many features with the other forms of myosi-tis recent developments have expanded our understanding of IBM so much that it is now considered the most common muscle disease in patients over 50 years.

Introduction

Commonly IBM, also known as 'sporadic inclusion body myositis' was only diagnosed when a patient with presumed polymyositis did not respond to therapy. Most investigators however would now agree that the features of IBM are distinctive enough to enable a primary diagnosis and not one of exclusion.

Presentation

It is the commonest acquired muscle disease occurring over the age of 50, affecting up to 300 people in the UK. Men are affected twice as commonly as women.

IBM typically presents in a middle-aged white male. The average time from onset of symptoms to diagnosis is 5 to 6 years. The patient is usually over 50 years. The history is usually one of insidious progressive weakness of both proximal (shoulder and hip) and distal (forearm and leg) muscles. Weakness can be asymmetric with particular involvement of the quadriceps (front of the thigh), iliopsoas (buttock muscles), biceps and triceps muscles. Finger flexor weakness and foot drop are seen. The patient may therefore complain of difficulty getting out of a chair, walking upstairs, stepping up onto a kerb and reaching above eye level. Atrophy (wasting) of muscles is common, as the disease process may have been ongoing for several years already by the time of diagnosis. Indeed severe wasting of the quadriceps for example may render the knee jerk absent raising the suspicion of a neurological disease. At this point the patient may complain of buckling of the knees.

Difficulty swallowing is a common occurrence. However the involvement of muscle in the heart is rare. IBM lacks the skin features of dermatomyositis but may be associated with a connective tissue disease in up to 15% of cases (Table 2).

Changes consistent with IBM have been described in childhood but this appears to be exceedingly rare.

The age of onset is some guide to how quickly the patient is likely to become debilitated. In patients who develop the disease in their forties, the average time from symptom onset to dependence on (Zimmer) frame walker is about 17 years. In those whose onset is in their seventies the interval is just over three years.

Table 2

Associated autoimmune diseases

- Systemic Lupus Erythematosus (SLE)
- Systemic Sclerosis (Scleroderma)
- Sjogren's syndrome (Dry eyes and mouth syndrome)

Diagnosis

Creatine Kinase

Any injury to skeletal muscle leads to muscle enzymes (proteins) leaking into the bloodstream. Thus elevated levels are valuable in detecting active muscle inflammation. Creatine kinase (CK) is the best studied muscle enzyme and the blood test to detect it is the most sensitive and commonly available for detecting skeletal muscle damage. Other tests are also useful but less-widely available (Table 3).

Table 3

Muscle enzymes released during muscle damage

- Aspartate Aminotransferase (AST)
- Alanine Aminotransferase (ALT)
- Aldolase
- Lactate Dehydrogenase (LDH)

These enzymes are not specific for muscle damage. Elevated levels of AST, ALT and LDH in particular raise the possibility of liver disease and have led to patients with myositis undergoing needless liver biopsies.

In IBM creatine kinase levels do not usually exceed 5 - 6 times normal and indeed can be within normal limits. The latter scenario is more likely with marked wasting.

Although no blood test is diagnostic of IBM up to 30% of patients have in their bloodstream "autoantibodies", proteins that react with different parts of the patients own cells. The significance of this is unclear.

Electromyogram

Needle Electromyography (EMG) is a sensitive but non-specific method of evaluating a muscle disorder. The EMG in myositis shows changes that can be interpreted by the electrophysiologist as being typical of myositis. However these findings are non-specific and do not hint at the cause of the myositis. Moreover mixed muscle and nerve signals may be present as a consequence of the regeneration of muscle fibres depending on the chronicity of the disease. Approximately 30% of IBM patients have EMG signs of axonal neuropathy, which means that the nerves have also been damaged. It is worth remembering that the focal nature of myositis can render a normal (false negative) EMG.

Muscle Biopsy

Muscle biopsy should be performed in all cases of suspected inflammatory myositis. Needle biopsy is less invasive than open biopsy but is prone to sampling error. EMG and Magnetic Resonance Imaging (MRI) can reduce this margin of error. MRI has the great advantage of scanning without using radiation. It is a very sensitive technique.

In acute myositis MRI shows focal increased signal intensities, especially on so-called T2-weighted (fat-suppressed) or STIR sequences. It has even been suggested that MRI can distinguish between polymyositis and inclusion body myositis. Thus by assessing the area of muscle with the highest signal intensity the most appropriate muscle can be selected for biopsy. Biopsy of a severely atrophied or non-inflamed muscle is not likely to be helpful.

What does the biopsy show in Inclusion Body Myositis?

The biopsy shows signs typical of many other types of inflammatory myositis but also features that are characteristic of IBM.

The common features are an abundance of white (inflammatory) cells with disruption of the muscle fibres (damaged or dead fibres, wasted fibres, and other areas showing regrowth of fibres). There may be evidence of inflammation within the capillaries supplying this particular muscle. There may be seen areas of scarring within the muscle.

Muscles are made up of small units called myofibrils, which form together into groups to form myofibres (fibres). In IBM (and polymyositis) the influx of white cells tends to be mainly around the lining of the myofibril rather than around the myofibre (dermato-myositis). The reason for this is not clear but it may be that there is more of a component of inflammation of the blood vessels (which lie along the myofibre) in dermatomyositis than in the other forms of myositis.

Most importantly in IBM are exclusively found the bodies that give the disorder its name – the inclusion bodies. These consist of vacuoles or cysts within the myofibril which are lined with dark-staining granules. Other features of IBM are seen on very high power microscopes and on electron microscopy. It is paramount that the laboratory preparing the biopsy specimens does so properly. The diagnosis of IBM can be missed if specimens are examined in paraffin-embedded sections only because the paraffin processing destroys the granules in the inclusion bodies making the vacuoles very difficult to see.

There is a familial form of IBM, so-called 'hereditary inclusion body myositis'. In these patients biopsy shows the typical inclusions but not the white cell infiltrate.

What causes IBM?

As it is classed as one of the 'Idiopathic Inflammatory Myositis' the cause of IBM is unknown. However recent new information has shed light on several aspects of IBM. Particular types of white cells, called T-cells, become activated by an as-yet-unknown factor. They remain activated for years after the onset of symptoms, leading to muscle cell breakdown.

Perhaps the breakdown of muscles is the primary event triggering a cascade of inflammatory responses. Proteins previously thought to occur only in the brains of Alzheimer's patients have been demonstrated within the IBM vacuoles. Does this suggest that IBM is a form of advanced ageing of muscles?

Infections have long been suspected as a cause of at least some cases of IBM. There is circumstantial evidence implicating viruses as possible trigger factors. Mumps and adenovirus, two very common viruses, have been isolated from IBM muscles in very rare, uncon-firmed reports.

Gene deletions in tiny intracellular particles called mitochondria have been demonstrated in isolated cases.

Treatment

The response to treatment is controversial and can be difficult to define. Periods of stabilisation lasting 3 to 6 months are seen in 25 to 50% of patients without therapy. Any course of therapy cannot be undertaken lightly. Close patient monitoring is required to assess subtle changes in muscle strength. Side effects to what can be toxic therapies must be watched for. Continuing therapeutic physical activity must be maintained and encouraged. Treatment thus requires a multi-disciplinary approach involving input form the rheumatology medical and nursing team, occupational therapists, physiotherapists and perhaps counselling services.

IBM's formidable reputation as a difficult disease is unfortunately well founded. Not every patient can expect to respond to therapy and indeed it may be unreasonable to expect any clear improvement in most patients. That said however it is now generally agreed that every patient deserves a therapeutic trial once IBM is diagnosed.

Therapy has focussed on suppressing the inflammatory response with a wide range of medications. Because of the inflammatory findings that are seen on biopsy most physicians will commence a trial of steroids, if only for a limited period of perhaps 3 months. There is evidence that steroids may however increase the numbers of vacuoles in the muscle fibrils, suggesting that IBM may primarily be a degenerative (wear-and-tear) disease with the inflammatory response playing a secondary role. Overall perhaps 40% of patients can expect an initial improvement with steroids, and perhaps more if treated simultaneously with another (immunosuppressive) drug.

Other medications that have been used with various levels of success include methotrexate, azathioprine and cyclosporin, alone or in combination. Chlorambucil was reported to be helpful in one refractory patient. Trials using cyclophosphamide and cyclosporin were perhaps too small to be conclusive.

Intravenous immunoglobulin (IVIg) has shown conflicting results and larger studies are needed. Case reports continue to appear of patients responding to various therapies e.g. mycophenolate.

Conclusion

Inclusion body myositis is an uncommon but significant disease. It is the most common muscle disease in patients over 50 years. The cause is probably multi-factorial. Onset is insidious. Diagnosis requires careful clinical assessment, blood tests, EMG and MRI and carefully selected biopsy. Recent developments have expanded our understanding of IBM. There remains a wide range of therapeutic options, all of which require the care of a committed multi-disciplinary team. More studies are required to elucidate the cause of this fascinating disease, which will ultimately lead to more effective treatment.

John McCarthy, ex-High School and University of Cork. Later Clinical Tutor/Research Fellow: University College Cork (1997).
I am still keen on Undergraduate teaching and plan a further research fellowship in the genetics of lupus and will later practice in Clinical Rheumatology as a Specialist.

References

Polymyositis, Dermatomyositis and Inclusion-Body Myositis
Dalakas MC, *NEJM* 1991, 325: 21; 1487 – 98

The Treatment of Inclusion-Body Myositis
Leff RL *et al*, *Medicine* 1993, 72: 4; 225 – 35

Myositis: Immunologic contributions to understanding Cause, Pathogenesis and Therapy
Plotz PH *et al*, *Annals of Internal Medicine* 1995, 122:9; 715 – 24

Magnetic resonance imaging criteria for distinguishing between Inclusion-Body Myositis and Polymyositis
Dion E *et al*, *J Rheumatol* 2002, 29: 9; 1897 – 906

Inclusion body myositis
Tawil R, Griggs RC, *Current Opinion in Rheumatology* 2002, 14: 6; 653 – 57

19

Lung Disease and Myositis

By Mona Manghani (MBChB, MRCP) and
Fiona Watt (BMed Sci, MBBS, MRCP)
Specialist Registrars in Rheumatology and General
Medicine, London Deanary 2005

Key Points

- Polymyositis and dermatomyositis are immune mediated disorders which target individual tissues within several organs.
- Skeletal muscle cells are a key target, but heart, lungs, joints, skin and kidneys may also be affected.
- Lung disease is often similar to that seen in other rheumatic disorders such as rheumatoid arthritis, scleroderma and systemic lupus erythematosus.

How can myositis affect the lungs?

There are two main ways myositis can affect the lung.

- Firstly, inflammation may occur within the substance of the lung as part of the immune process in myositis – this is called **interstitial lung disease** or ILD.
- Secondly, the myositis may affect the muscles that help you breath, resulting in weak respiratory muscles. In addition to this medications used in the treatment of myositis may affect the lungs.

Interstitial lung disease and myositis

Interstitial lung disease forms the biggest group of lung conditions that may affect someone with myositis. ILD may develop with the first attack of myositis, precede the muscle disease by several years or develop following the diagnosis. This is why physicians need to be alert to the risk at all stages of the disease.

ILD may present in three different ways:

- asymptomatic disease (where patients will be unaware there is a problem with their lungs),
- chronic disease (where breathing problems may come on slowly, and may be a long-lasting feature),
- acute disease (where sudden onset of breathing problems may be severe and sometimes life-threatening, but may respond well to aggressive therapy).

This last type is extremely unusual in the myositis patient group.

How is the lung affected?
Interstitial (or interstitium) refers to a normally tiny space between cells containing fluid. The interstitium in the lung is within the respiratory membrane. This membrane is an interface made up of tiny bubble like sacs (alveoli) at the ends of the airways and the associated wall. Oxygen has to pass through this membrane and into tiny blood vessels. Poisonous gases such as carbon dioxide pass out in a reverse mechanism into the exhaled air. This process is essential to allow the body to gain enough oxygen to pass to all the tissues of the body. Because of the enormous surface area of this membrane (approximately 100 square metres in the normal adult), we can achieve this process very efficiently. However, any process that enlarges the interstitial space, and so thickens the respiratory membrane increases the distance over which oxygen has to travel, making this process less efficient. If severe enough, interstitial disease within the lung can restrict both the ability of the alveoli to absorb oxygen and may also restrict the volume and movements of the lung, causing the symptoms of lung disease.

Are there different types of interstitial lung disease?
Different types of interstitial lung disease exist, and within the myositis group there are a variety of different patterns. They will often cause the same symptoms, but are distinguishable on detailed X ray testing or by taking minute biopsy samples of the lung. The type of pattern can help your physician assess how severe the disease is likely to become and how aggressive to be with any drug treatment.

Current terminology is complicated and often confusing, as the names of these conditions are often being re-classified. Those seen within the myositis patient group include cryptogenic organizing pneumonitis (COP), non specific interstitial pneumonitis (NSIP) and usual interstitial pneumonitis (UIP). NSIP is the commonest type seen in polymyositis.

Each of these conditions is associated with the passage of immune cells into the interstitial layer of the lung, which cause inflammation at this site. This inflammatory change can ultimately lead to lung fibrosis - that is scarring of the lung, which leads to permanent changes which are not reversible. It is important to identify any pre-cursor of inflammation within the lung, which may respond to treatment, thereby preventing fibrosis. This is the main objective of disease management.

Interstitial lung disease in other rheumatic conditions

Interstitial lung disease may also occur in different rheumatic conditions such as systemic lupus erthematosus (SLE), Sjogren's disease, scleroderma, rheumatoid arthritis, mixed connective tissue disease and overlap syndromes. The ILD that can occur in SLE and scleroderma are of the NSIP type.

In the latter, patients may have clinical features of more than one connective tissue disease. For example a patient with an SLE/myositis overlap syndrome may have typical lupus features and marked muscle weakness. Specific antibodies have been closely linked to the various groups of overlap syndromes. Isolating these autoantibodies in the blood of patients not only aid in the diagnosis of the condition, but also help in identifying those patients who are at an increased likelihood of developing interstitial lung disease.

Other lung diseases and myositis

Respiratory muscle weakness

Myositis causes muscle weakness, which can affect the respiratory muscles. These are the muscles of the rib cage and the diaphragm, which allow us to take breaths of air and also to perform important manoeuvres such as coughing to prevent aspiration – literally things 'going down the wrong way'. Rarely, respiratory muscle weakness may be severe enough that a patient may need oxygen or full ventillatory support, which is usually provided on an intensive care unit (ICU), often with the patient asleep.

Aspiration pneumonia

A combination of weakness of muscles of swallowing in certain myositis patients and a poor cough reflex can lead to aspiration, particularly when the disease is new and untreated. This can lead to pneumonia, because bacteria from the mouth and gut are passed into the lungs. The potential for this risk can be assessed by medical staff and speech therapists, and by use of pulmonary function testing (see below). If there is concern about risk of aspiration, feeding may have to be given temporarily via a naso-gastric tube, directly into the stomach, while the myositis is treated.

Myositis drugs and the lungs

Powerful drugs such as steroids and other disease-modifying drugs which suppress the immune system are usually required to treat a patient's myositis effectively. In more severe disease, high dose chemotherapy drugs may be needed. The side effect is the reduction of the normal immune response to common bacterial infections. Chest infections and pneumonia become a major concern in this patient group, because patients are less mobile, less able to take a deep breath and clear secretions, and may also have underlying lung disease. Careful monitoring and chest physiotherapy have an important role in prevention of pneumonia which requires antibiotics and hospital care if it develops.

Occasionally, certain drugs used in myositis treatment can cause lung problems as a direct side effect. Methotrexate, which is a drug often used in polymyositis and dermatomyositis has a low risk itself of causing inflammation within the lung (pneumonitis) and lung fibrosis. All patients starting this treatment should therefore always have a chest X ray to check for underlying lung disease. The likelihood of this side effect is increased in smokers, who should be advised to stop. It may also be associated with increasing length of treatment with methotrexate.

Who gets lung disease in myositis?

Studies estimate that between 5% and 40% of patients with myositis develop interstitial lung disease. This is usually diagnosed after testing (discussed in the next section) and includes those with no symptoms of lung disease. The rate seems to vary between populations, with more lung involvement in Japanese myositis populations than U.S populations, although this could be explained by the differing techniques used to identify lung disease in different studies.

Clues from my disease

Joint pains and fever seem to be far more common in patients who suffer from ILD. There is no particular link between ILD and the rare cases of malignancy causing myositis. Lung disease can be associated with a shorter life expectancy, particularly if the disease is severe. Lung disease seems to affect similar proportions of patients with dermatomyositis and polymyositis.

Clues from my test results

The isolation of certain auto-antibodies within the blood may be associated with an increased risk of developing interstitial lung disease. The anti-synthetase antibodies, of which anti-Jo-1 is the commonest, have a strong association with interstitial lung disease. Patients with these antibodies often have features of myositis, arthritis, Raynaud's phenomenon, ILD and scaling, cracked hands (Mechanic's hands). Anti-Mi-2 antibodies occur more commonly in dermatomyositis and are not associated with ILD. There have been small numbers of patients with dermatomyositis with classical skin features in the absence of myositis, who develop very aggressive interstitial lung disease. Such patients may have a higher ratio of CD4 T cells in the blood. (See *What is Myositis?* Chapter 2)

Myositis-associated autoantibodies are found in the overlap syndromes of myositis with SLE , scleroderma or mixed connective tissue. Anti-Ku are found in the polymyositis/scleroderma overlap as is anti-PM-Scl. Anti-U1-RNP occurs in polymyositis/SLE/mixed connective tissue disease overlap.

In all of these conditions the patient may present with symptoms of lung disease first, and other organs such as muscle or skin may be affected at a later date. Therefore it is important to always keep an open mind in regards to the underlying rheumatic condition. The auto-antibody profile is important and helps in the process of the ultimate diagnosis.

Do we understand the cause of interstitial lung disease?

Several factors are thought to have a role in the cause of interstitial lung disease in myositis, although a definite cause remains unclear. Jo-1 antibodies have been found in samples taken from the lungs of some patients, suggesting that they may be associated with causing disease, possibly by triggering immune cells to cause inflammatory damage. Infections are thought to be potentially important in allowing lung disease to develop, and those implicated include Epstein-Barr virus (glandular fever or infectious mononucleosis), cytomegalovirus and even hepatitis C virus, although a definite link has not been proven. The hypothesis is that these infections trigger an immune response in a genetically susceptible individual – similar to sowing a seed in a previously ploughed field.

How will my doctor know if I have lung disease?

Certain symptoms and test results will suggest to a physician that a patient with myositis may be developing lung disease. The possibility of asymptomatic disease and the importance of detecting it means your physician will often request many of the tests below as routine surveillance.

Symptoms associated with lung disease

These tend to be similar in the different types of lung disease. Shortness of breath is initially likely to be when exerting oneself, and is usually gradual in onset. Because myositis itself often limits what people can do, this presentation of lung disease may often be 'masked' – for example, if someone is only able to walk ten yards, then the disease will have to be relatively more severe to be noticeable, compared with someone who is able to walk for two miles.

A dry, non-productive cough can often be associated with the development of lung disease. However, it should be borne in mind that by far the commonest cause of dry cough is still colds and chest infections. Rarely, interstitial lung disease can cause chest pains. They are classically sharp and worse on deep breathing ('pleuritic chest pain'). Advice should always be sought from a physician as to the cause of chest pains, because of the number of other potential causes.

It should be noted that other conditions caused by myositis can also cause breathing symptoms, particularly heart involvement. Although rare, cardiac failure or rhythm disturbance can produce shortness of breath, as can involvement of the respiratory muscles.

Signs of lung disease
Signs to your physician that interstitial lung disease may be developing include reduced inflation of the chest and fine crackles at the base of the lungs when listening with a stethoscope. They will usually listen to your chest as part of your routine check-up. However, these signs may be absent, particularly in early disease.

Tests for lung disease in myositis
- *Chest X- ray*

A chest X- ray will be performed routinely by your physician. In lung disease, this can sometimes show shadowing, usually at the base of the lungs, suggesting lung fibrosis. The diaphragms may be higher than normal, also indicating a lung problem. However, early interstitial lung disease may not show up on a chest X- ray and so other tests are required to exclude it.

- *Pulmonary function testing*

Pulmonary function testing (PFTs) are performed by a trained respiratory technician. They do not hurt in any way, and involve blowing into a tube connected to a machine. They measure lung volumes, which may be reduced in interstitial lung disease. They also measure transfer factor, which is a measure of how efficiently gases are being transferred across the respiratory membrane in the lung. In interstitial disease, the thickness of the membrane increases, which will cause a reduction in the transfer factor. This is usually expressed as a percentage of the value expected for a healthy person of the same age and height. This is important, as it is a sensitive way of detecting an interstitial lung problem and also monitoring its progress, for example in response to treatment. Those with a transfer factor of less than 55% may start to develop problems with increasing levels of the poisonous gas carbon dioxide in the blood, particularly if they also have respiratory muscle weakness. This can cause fatigue and can be tested for by taking an arterial blood gas sample.

• *Computerized tomography*

More sophisticated X- ray tests now exist. Thin section 'high resolution' computerized axial tomography ('CT scanning' or CAT scanning) is the most effective way of detailing any changes going on within the lungs of those patients with myositis. The scans need to be interpreted by a radiologist and can also help to classify the disease. CT scans may also be used to track progress although, given the significant X- ray exposure involved, they are always kept to a minimum.

'Ground glass' changes may suggest inflammatory change, which may respond to treatment. Changes in fibrosis can also be detected. When these changes are severe, leading to obvious loss of lung tissue, it may be described as 'honey-combing' of the lung, because of the pattern on CT.

• *Blood tests*

These have already been discussed

None of these tests will detect all patients with interstitial lung disease. Early disease may not be visualised on CT, and transfer factor is often the best way of detecting if disease is present (although other factors may influence transfer factor, and your physician will need to interpret this test carefully). Occasionally, particularly in rapidly progressive disease, specialist centres may wish to perform other tests such as bronchoalveolar lavage (washings of the lung, performed during a telescope test of the airways) or even lung biopsy to aid in treatment decisions.

What treatments are there for lung disease in myositis?

Polymyositis and dermatomyositis are rare disorders, and interstitial lung disease includes a number of different disease processes, which only affect some PM/DM patients. As a result there is no strong trial evidence on the use of drugs in myositis lung disease. Most of the evidence comes from interstitial lung disease in other conditions.

The treatment of lung disease is very much a part of the treatment of the overall condition. The mainstay is steroids, usually with other drugs such as azathioprine and cyclosporin A. Many patients may already be receiving these drugs for their myositis. In this situation, and in the presence of mild interstitial disease, it may be a question of continuing normal therapy while watching tests to check that the lung condition is not deteriorating.

In more severe lung disease, or in disease which is rapidly progressive, options may include high dose intravenous drips of methylprednisolone repeated over three days, as this has immediate immunosuppressive and anti inflammatory effects. In addition, drugs such as cyclophosphamide may be used. This is a chemotherapeutic agent found to be effective in the treatment of some inflammatory lung disease. It may be given as a tablet, or more usually as a course of once monthly infusions into the vein, over a six month period.

Trials have shown favourable results with cyclophosphamide in scleroderma lung disease. NSIP is the most common type of interstitial lung disease in scleroderma, as it is in PM/DM lung disease, and there is substantial evidence that cyclophosphamide is better than any other immunosuppressants in preserving lung function and survival. Japanese and European studies have also shown that cyclosporin A in combination with azathioprine and cyclophosphamide have also been beneficial. Immunosuppressants are powerful drugs which have potential serious side effects, requiring careful assessment and discussion between the physician and the patient before they are used.

Current studies using Bosentan, (an inhibitor of endothelin -1), have shown anti-fibrotic activity both in the laboratory and in an international study in scleroderma patients with interstitial lung disease. In addition other anti-fibrotic agents are also being studied.

As previously discussed, the degree of inflammation, as opposed to fibrosis, will impact on how much a patient may respond to any of these treatments, as they can be seen as strongly anti-inflammatory, although working in different ways.

Conclusions

- Important lung conditions that may affect a patient with myositis are defined- in particular interstitial lung disease.

- Around a third of patients may be affected, although many may be asymptomatic because of the limitations of their muscle disease.

- Close monitoring for the development of this important and often insidious manifestation of myositis disease is important, but an awareness of potential symptoms in patients is also essential.

- In those patients who present with respiratory symptoms of ILD initially, it is important to keep an open mind in regards to the underlying rheumatic condition, as many conditions are associated with ILD.

- Serial lung function tests and CT scans are used to assess progress and response to treatment.

- Treatment options and current studies are discussed.

Mona Manghani and Fiona Watts are specialist registrars in rheumatology. Mona is currently on a Sports Medicine fellowship in Sydney and Fiona is studying for a PhD in London.

20

Dysphagia

by Theresa Curry

S peech professionals believe that as many as 80 per cent of myositis patients may have either temporary or permanent problems with swallowing, ranging from very mild and treatable to severe. It's not surprising, says Don Barbarino, staff speech pathologist for Forbes Regional Hospital in Monroeville, PA: "More than 30 different muscles are involved in this process. Most of us don't give swallowing a thought – it's over in seconds, and works as naturally as breathing in and out."

For the myositis patient with weakened face, tongue and throat muscles, the process is much more complicated, and weak muscles can interfere in any of the steps of this deceptively complex process. Barbarino says that weak muscles can change the process as you open your mouth and chew your food; as your tongue moves it to the back of your mouth; as you block off your windpipe (larynx) to allow the food to go down the right path (pharynx) to your stomach; and as the slight contractions of your oesophagus move the food to your stomach.

Signs that muscle weakness may be interfering with your swallowing are many, and may be so subtle that you don't pay much attention. Early in the process you may find that you can't form the food into a mass (called a "bolus") on your tongue. You may find that it's taking a long time to get the food to the back of your mouth, that it's slipping down your throat before you're ready, or that you're not able to close off your larynx, causing what we describe as "food going down the wrong way". The danger in this is that particles of food will lodge in your lungs, leading to aspiration pneumonia. Reflux or heartburn may be an early sign that swallowing has been affected.

Other signs, said Barbarino, are lip weakness and drooling, facial droop, a feeling of weakness in your tongue, aspirating food into your nose, coughing or choking while you eat, or having to clear your throat a lot. Also watch out for the feeling of having a lump in your throat, tightness in your chest, pain when swallowing, or shortness of breath after you eat. If you're actually aspirating food, you may also find you're sneezing, burping, or hiccuping a great deal at mealtime. Tell your doctor right away if you have any of these symptoms.

There are a number of ways that you and your doctor can manage this troublesome complication of myositis. Your physician may want to use a team approach, perhaps referring you to a speech pathologist, a gastroenterologist, an otolaryngologist, a dietician, or an occupational therapist. You may find that other members of your family will get involved, too, as you learn what works for you in the management of this problem. There are some diagnostic tools and tests that will allow your physician to observe your swallow, or he or she may make a diagnosis and treatment recommendation based solely on your symptoms.

Some techniques for improving your swallowing are quite simple. Barbarino recommends that even patients who don't have any dysphagia symptoms sit upright, chew thoroughly, avoid distractions and avoid eating after 8pm. You may work with a speech pathologist to change the way you hold your head, for example, positioning your chin at different angles, or you may discover that you only have trouble with certain consistencies. It may help to only eat foods of the same consistency at one time. You may find that it helps to eat more slowly, or eat smaller portions.

The same medications that improve overall myositis symptoms may improve swallowing problems. In a recent paper, The Myositis Association Medical Advisory Board Member, Dr. Chester Oddis described a study in which three patients – two with dermatomyositis and one polymyositis patient with complications – had dramatic and rapid improvement with IVIg leading to improved swallowing within two weeks. However, Dr. Oddis observed, corticosteroids were also being used, making the contribution of IVIg difficult to judge. Dr. Oddis also found that patients with chronic contractions (more common in IBM), accompanied by a blocking sensation and cough with swallowing, often responded to myotomy, a simple surgical procedure that 'stretches' part of the throat.

Some people have expressed satisfaction with feeding tubes, a step that isn't as drastic and final as you might believe. It can be a practical and very helpful way to avoid the danger of choking and aspiration pneumonia. Dr. Todd Levine, a Phoenix neurologist who has a number of myositis patients, recommends this for his patients BEFORE they experience pneumonia or a serious choking problem. The tube enters your stomach through a small button and can be used for supplemental feedings. Patients may continue to eat foods that they tolerate and to join their families and friends for part of dinner or a restaurant meal, and they may have the tube removed when symptoms disappear.

General Recommendations for Swallowing:

- Sit upright while eating and 1-2 hours after eating. This position will help direct the food toward your stomach.

- Try to eat when you are not fatigued. Chewing and swallowing will be more efficient if you eat when you are rested.

- Take smaller bites of food and smaller sips of liquid. Smaller bites and sips are easier to manage in the mouth and throat.

- Take one bite or sip at a time. Be sure that your mouth is clear before taking another bite or sip.

- Increase sensory input you get from your food. By eating foods served either hot or cold, foods with texture, and foods that are flavourful, sensory information travels from your mouth to the brain and signals to your brain to begin the swallow.

- During mealtimes, focus your attention on eating. Try to avoid distractions such as television.

- Drink plenty of water and liquids. Your body functions best when properly hydrated. Cold liquids are recommended, as they tend to stimulate the swallow. One suggestion is to blend water or juice with ice in a blender to make a cold, slushy drink. Additionally, taking enough water will thin out your secretions and help to combat thick, stringy saliva.

- If mealtimes are taking too long, try eating six small meals per day rather than three large ones. Eating a smaller amount of food at each meal is less tiring.

- Avoid foods that are most difficult to chew and swallow and foods that are difficult to control in the mouth.

- Maintain good oral hygiene. Research shows that this prevents aspiration pneumonia in individuals with swallowing disorders.

DYSPHAGIA GLOSSARY

DEGLUTITION (*DEE gloo TISH un*) – the act of swallowing

DYSPHAGIA (*dis FAY jee yah*) – difficulty swallowing; difficulty moving food or liquids from mouth to stomach

LARYNGEAL (*le RIN jee uhl*) penetration – foreign material enters the larynx (vestibule, windpipe) but remains above the vocal chords

LARYNX (*LARE inks*) – muscle and cartilage that holds the vocal chords

PHARYNX (*FARE inks*) – area leading from the mouth and nose to the larynx and esophagus

OESOPHAGUS (*i SOF uh gus*) – tube that passes food from the pharynx to the stomach

ASPIRATION (*AS puh RAY shen*) – foreign material enters the larynx and below the vocal chords toward the lungs

STRICTURE (*STRIK cher*) – narrowing of a tube

ACHALASIA (*A kuh LAY shuh*) – failure to relax; persistent contraction.

Theresa Curry is the Communications Director for The Myositis Association. This article first appeared in the March 2003 edition of the TMA newsletter, 'The Outlook'.

SECTION FIVE

Resources

How to claim Disability Living Allowance

compiled by Janet Horton 2005

1. Keep a diary for at least a week showing:-

    a) how far you can walk without severe discomfort.

    b) how long it takes you to walk that distance.

    c) record the sort of hands on personal care you need, how often and for how long on each occasion.

2. Request a DLA claim pack from the Department of Work and Pensions.

When it arrives, go through it and make notes on a separate piece of paper about what you would put in the spaces provided.

THEN – MOST IMPORTANTLY OF ALL – go to your local Citizen's Advice Bureau, Welfare Rights or Disability Agency such as DIAL for help with the completion of the form.

This advice is the same for Incapacity Benefit.

Useful
Resources

No responsibility can be taken for the services offered. This list is for information on where you can seek further help.

MYOSITIS SUPPORT GROUPS

Myositis Support Group UK
146 Newtown Road, Woolston, Southampton SO19 9HR
023 8044 9708 Fax: 023 8039 6402
Email: msg@myositis.org.uk
www.myositis.org.uk

The Myositis Association
1233 20th St. NW, Suite 402, Washington, DC 20036
P: (202) 887-0088 F: (202) 466-8940
www. tma@myositis.org

RELATED GROUPS

Arthritis Research Campaign
St. Mary's Gate, Chesterfield, Derbyshire S41 7TD
01246 558033 Email: info@arc.org.uk www.arc.org.uk
The UK's fourth biggest medical research charity which funds research into all types of arthritis and musculoskeletal disease including myositis. It also produces patient literature, including a free booklet, 'Polymyositis and Dermatomyositis.'

Muscular Dystrophy Campaign
7-11 Prescott Place, London SW4 6BS
0207 720 8055

DISABILITY

Easifuel – gadget to aid when filling up with fuel at a service station.
Available for £2.99 incl. p&p but you can try before you buy.
17 Chapter Road, London SE17 3ES 020 7582 1117

Handybar – aids getting in or out of a vehicle
www.mobilityconversions.co.uk

The Disabled Driver's Motor Club
www.ddmc.org.uk 01832 734 724

House of Bath 'Health and Self'
www.houseofbath.co.uk 08701 606 101

Homecraft is the UK's largest distributor of Daily Living, Therapy and
Paediatric products. www.homecraft-rolyan.com

Disability Exhibitions
Email: events@disabilitynorth.org.uk

Ricability is the trading name of the Research Institute for Consumer
Affairs (RICA). A national research charity dedicated to providing
independent information of value to disabled and older consumers.
www.ricability.org.uk

Disability Now Online
The UK's biggest selling disability related newspaper.
www.disabilitynow.org.uk

SKIN CAMOUFLAGE

British Association of Skin Camouflage, South Park Road,
Macclesfield, Cheshire SK11 6FP 01625 871129
Email: basc9@hotmail.com www.skin.camouflage.net

COUNSELLING SERVICES

Association of Child Psychotherapists
020 8458 1609

British Association for Counselling
01788 550899 or www.bac.co.uk

British Association of Psychotherapists
020 8452 9823 or www.bcp.org.uk

Centre for Stress Management
www.managingstress.com

Directory of Internet Mental Health Resources
www.mentalhealth.com

International Stress Management Association
07000 780 430 or www.isma.org.uk

Mind
www.mind.org.uk or write to Mind Publications, Granta House,
15-19 Broadway, London E15 4BQ. Enclose an A4 stamped
addressed envelope.

National Register of Hypnotherapists and Psychotherapists
01282 716 839 or www.nrhp.co.uk

Relate
01788 573 241 or www.relate.org.uk

UK Council of Psychotherapy
020 7436 3002 or www.psychotherapy.org.uk

HERBAL AND NUTRITIONAL THERAPY

British Association of Nutritional Therapists (BANT)
0870 606 1284 or www.bant.org.uk

Food and Mood Project
www.foodandmood.org

General Council and Register of Consultant Herbalists
01792 655 886 or www.aromacaring.co.uk

General Council and Register of Naturopaths
01458 840 072 or www.naturopathy.org.uk

National Institute of Medical Herbalists
01392 426 022 or www.btinternet.com/-nimh/

RELAXATION

Autogenic Therapy (BAFATT)
020 7837 8833
c/o The Royal London Homeopathic Hospital, NHS Trust,
Great Ormond Street, London WC1N 3HR. Send an SAE.

British Wheel of Yoga
01529 306 851 or www.bwy.org.uk

Pilates Foundation
020 8281 5087 pr www.pilatesfoundation.com

School of Meditation
020 7603 6116 or www.schoolofmeditation.org

Society of Teachers of The Alexander Technique
020 7284 3338 or www.stat.org.uk

T'ai Chi (Quigong)
0161 929 4485 or www.qimagazine.com

National T'ai Chi Chuan Association
020 8556 6393 or www.taichifinder.co.uk

COMPLEMENTARY THERAPIES

Acupuncture and Osteopathic Association
020 7834 1012

Association of Reflexologists
0070 567 3320 or www.aor.org.uk

Bach Flower Remedies
The Bach Centre 01491 834 678 or www.bachcentre.com

British Acupuncture Council
020 8735 0400 or www.acupuncture.org.uk

British Homeopathic Association
020 7566 7800 or www.trusthomeopathy.org

Council for Complementary and Alternative Medicine (CCAM)
0207 724 9103 or www.drlockie.com

Complementary Medical Association
0208305 9571 or www.the-cma.org.uk

Institute for Complementary Medicine
0207237 5165 or www.icmedicine.co.uk

USEFUL PUBLICATIONS

Not Dead Yet
Dr Robert Buckman talks about his dermatomyositis in this autobiography available through bookfinder.com or amazon.com (Doubleday Canada)

Sick and Tired of Feeling Sick and Tired
Paul J. Donoghue Ph.D., Mary E. Siegel Ph.D. (Norton 1994)

Coping with Prednisone
Eugenia Zukerman and Julie R. Ingelfinger, M.D.
(St. Martin's Griffin 1997)

Coping with a Myositis Disease
James R. Kilpatrick (Kilpatrick Publishing Company 2000)

Broken Glass and All
An account of the author's battle with polymyositis and his cure in Montreal using naturopathic medicine and Homeopathy.
A.D. Squitieri, PO Box 605, Fulton, N.Y. 13069 USA
www.adswordwright.com

E For Additives
Maurice Hanssen with Jill Marsden (Thorsons 1988)

The Vitamin Bible
Earl Mindell (Arlington Books 1982)

The Herb Bible
Earl Mindell (Vermilion 1994)

Complete Nutrition
Dr Michael Sharon (Prion 1997)

Healing Foods
Miriam Polunin (Dorling Kindersley 1997)

Foods for Mind and Body
Michael van Straten (Harper Collins 1997)

The Complete Guide to Food Allergy and Intolerance
Dr Jonathan Brostoff and Linda Gamlin (Bloomsbury 1992)

The Food Bible
Judith Wills (Quadrille Publishing Ltd 2002)

The Oracle Diet
Michael van Straten (Kyle Cathie Limited 2002)

The Food Doctor
Vicki Edgson and Ian Marber (Collins and Brown 1999)

Cooking Without
Barbara Cousins (Thorsons 2000)

Vegetarian Cooking Without
Barbara Cousins (Thorsons 2000)

Super Juice
Michael van Straten (Mitchell Beazley 1999)

Food and Juice for Health
(Hamlyn 2002)

Camouflage

by Janelle Jones

I have Juvenile Dermatomyositis. I was treated by Great Ormond Street Hospital in London from diagnosis at the age of 7 years until I was 16 years old. I have the typical heliotrope rash predominately on my face.

During my teens, I became very self conscious and was often called cruel names such as "spotty dog", which was very hurtful!

I began to experiment with cosmetics from about the age of 15. I was also referred to the Red Cross for advice about camouflage products.

The outcome initially was not too successful. Yes, the camouflage covered the rash on my face but I felt too young to wear what I considered to be such 'thick' makeup. I still found people would stare at me and I was not comfortable with it.

I continued to try other products over the years; I probably spent a fortune on cosmetics!

I joined the Myositis Support group about 6 years ago and while I was at an AGM meeting I picked up an article about the British Association of Skin Camouflage.

I subsequently joined and contacted a local practitioner who gave me some advice about using camouflage products and also matched my skin tone to recommend a particular product which I was then able to get on prescription from my doctor.

I have been using this product ever since, with good results and a boost to my self confidence.

This experience made me realise that there must be a lot of people with skin problems who like me had found it difficult to obtain advice.

In August 2003, I decided to train as a Camouflage practitioner and attended the excellent course that the British Association of Skin Camouflage runs twice a year.

I was impressed by the range of products available and the many skin conditions that it will disguise, also enriching and giving confidence to the people who use these products.

Being a member of BASC doesn't cost much. You will receive regular newsletters and invitations to many courses and meetings. The BASC will be able to advise people about a practitioner in your area.

For further advice contact:
Mary Thorp, BASC Executive Office, BASC Resources for Business LTD, South Park Road, Macclesfield, Cheshire SK11 6FP www.skin.camouflage.net Email basc9@hotmail.com
Tel: 01625 871129

Glossary
of terms

ALANINE AMINOTRANSFERASE (**ALT** or glutamic pyruvic transaminase) – Enzyme produced by the liver in response to inflammation.

ALDOLASE – Enzyme produced by the liver in response to inflammation.

AMYOPATHIC DERMATOMYOSITIS – A dermatomyositis-like illness with skin associated pathology (e.g. rash) but no muscle weakness or pain.

ANAEMIA – Deficiency in red blood cells in the bloodstream. Patients on methotrexate require folic acid (folate) supplements to avoid anaemia.

ANTIBODY – A specialized protein circulating in the blood conferring immunity to disease (e.g. antibodies are produced by the body following vaccination and these then fight off disease) – see autoantibodies and antigen.

ARD – Autoimmune Rheumatic Diseases.

ASPARTATE AMINOTRANSFERASE (AST) – Enzyme produced by the liver in response to inflammation.

ANA – Anti-nuclear Antibody. These antibodies are produced when by 'B' lymphocytes or B cells produce antibodies against a number of different structures associated with the nucleus of cells. For example, in lupus, the ANA is often against double stranded DNA itself. In others it is against other DNA-associated structures such as RNA, nucleosomes or other proteins/enzymes in the cell. Patients with raised levels of ANA may have a number of possible diseases including myositis, SLE (systemic lupus erythematosus), and other immune mediated connective tissue diseases including rheumatoid arthritis.

ANTIGEN – The part of a protein molecule that can be recognised by immune cells. Antibodies recognise and bind to antigens on the surface of viruses, bacteria and in the case of autoimmune diseases, tissues.

ASPIRATION – Inhalation of food or drink etc. into the lungs.

ASPIRATION PNEUMONIA – Infection of the lungs caused by food/drink being inhaled.

AUTOANTIBODIES – Antibodies that are produced inappropriately that are directed against self or normal tissues/cells. For example, ANA, Anti-DNA, Anti-Jo-1, Anti-Mi, Anti-SRP. Patients with anti-Jo-1 frequently have interstitial lung disease, whereas patients with anti-SRP may have a less aggressive disease.

AUTOIMMUNE – Autoimmune illnesses occur when the body reacts to it's own tissues. The disease is caused either by antibodies being made by 'B' lymphocytes (white cells in the blood) against the body's own tissues, or certain other white blood cells ('macrophages, T' cells, natural killer (NK) cells) attack the tissues. In most autoimmune illnesses, the reason why this occurs is not known, however some people may be more susceptible than others due to a polygenetic effect which also requires a multifactorial environmental set of triggers. Patients with one autoimmune illness e.g. myositis, will sometimes have others (e.g. thyroid problems, coeliac disease), and the incidence of these types of disorder are more frequent in family members, though myositis in the same family is not recognised.

'B' CELLS – A sub-set of white blood cells (lymphocytes) whose main function is to produce antibodies, normally against diseases such as viruses or bacteria. In autoimmune diseases, 'B' cells are out of control in terms of producing antibodies, which can damage normal tissues such as muscles.

'T' CELLS – Like 'B' cells, these cells are also white blood cells (lymphocytes). However, these cells do not produce antibodies, but can either help 'B' cells recognise foreign agents such as viruses or bacteria, or actively kill such agents (NK or natural killer cells). In some autoimmune diseases, 'T' cells are often responsible for attacking or provoking an attack on normal tissues.

BARIUM SWALLOW – An X-ray test to determine the ability to swallow. Barium appears white on X-ray and will show up problems in swallowing.

BIOLOGIC – Agents made by a biological process (non-chemical) used to prevent or treat disease (e.g. Immunoglobulin (IgG, IVIg, monoclonal antibodies etc.)

BIOPSY – Removal of a small amount of tissue for examination.

BUFFALO HUMP – Accumulation of fat at the back of the neck.

CALCINOSIS – The abnormal presence of calcium (chalky deposits) in tissues.

CALCIFICATION – The process of calcium deposition into tissues.

CAPILLARIES – Very small blood vessels which join the ends of the arteries to the commencement of the veins.

COELIAC DISEASE – This is another autoimmune disease where patients cannot tolerate gluten in their diet. This disease is characterised by a chronic gastro-intestinal disturbances, and can become serious if left undiagnosed. Patients diagnosed with one autoimmune diseases often have others as well (see Thyroid).

CONTRACTURE – The shortening of muscles or tendons which prevents the associated joints from moving freely.

CPK (OR CK) LEVEL – Creatine Phosphokinase – an enzyme found in skeletal muscle. When the CPK level is substantially elevated, it usually indicates injury (e.g. Myositis). A simple blood test can measure levels of creatine phosphokinase. A value of between 25 and 200 is usually regarded as normal (although hospitals vary greatly in the levels given as being within normal limits), and levels can escalate into the thousands in patients with active disease. Hence a myositis 'flare' is often diagnosed by a sharp increase in CK or CPK values.

CRP OR C-REACTIVE PROTEIN – A factor found in the blood produced by the liver. High levels indicate inflammation occurring somewhere in the body.

CYTOKINES – Soluble molecules produced by cells of the immune system in order to communicate with one another.

CYTOTOXIC – Poisonous to cells. Cytotoxic medicines can be used to kill unwanted cells or tissues (e.g. in cancer therapy).

DYSPHAGIA – Difficulty in swallowing.

EFFICACY – The effectiveness of a treatment/medicine.

ELECTROMYOGRAPH (EMG) – A diagnostic machine that detects the electrical activity of functioning skeletal muscle. Used to diagnose neuro-muscular disorders.

ENDOSCOPE – A telescope/camera that can be used to look inside a hollow organ (e.g. down a patients throat).

ENZYME – A protein that triggers chemical reactions in the body (see CPK).

ESR (Erythrocyte Sedimentation Rate) – Erythrocytes are the red cells in blood. When you get ill, the constituents of blood plasma (the clear sus-pension fluid in blood) alters, with new proteins (or acute phase reactants) entering the plasma. These proteins bind non-specifically to the red-blood cells. When a blood sample is taken, doctors can calculate how long it takes for the red-blood cells to settle out in a test-tube (mm of red-blood cells per hour). Blood cells with protein attached will settle out faster than 'normal' blood cells. Thus an elevated ESR means that you are unwell, but it can't predict exactly what with.

FAMILIAL – Linked to a family but not necessarily genetically linked.

FIBROSIS – Replacement of normal tissue with scar tissue.

"FIRST-LINE" TREATMENT – The standard treatment tried first by the majority of doctors.

FLARE – If myositis has been in remission, but returns unexpectedly, this is known as a 'flare'.

FOLIC ACID (FOLATE) – A vitamin of the B complex required for nor-mal production of red blood cells. Used in the treatment of anaemia. Occurs naturally in liver, kidneys, green leafy vegetables, dried beans and mushrooms.

GENERIC – an off-patent medicine made by a company other than the medicine producer. Cheaper than the original, but sometimes not as effective due to formulation differences.

GOTTRON'S SIGN – Redness of the knuckles with raised, scaly eruptions/lesions.

HELIOTROPE RASH – Blue/purple discoloration of the upper eyelids with swelling.

IDIOPATHIC – Arising spontaneously or from an obscure or unknown cause (e.g. idiopathic inflammatory myopathy).

IMMUNE RESPONSE – The response by the body to "foreign" material (transplant or infection).

IMMUNOGLOBULINS – Antibodies.

IMMUNOMODULATION – Alteration of the immune response by treatment etc.

IMMUNOSUPPRESSANTS – Prescribed medicines/drugs which aim to suppress the immune system. These include prednisone, prednisolone, methotrexate, Imuran, cyclosporin, cyclophosphamide, tacrolimus etc.

INTERLEUKINS – Soluble substances produced by lymphocytes, macrophages, and monocytes that regulate the cell-mediated immune system.

INTERSTITIAL LUNG DISEASE – Inflammation leading to fibrosis (scarring) of the lung tissues.

INTRAVENOUS – A method of administering treatments directly into the vein.

LACTATE DEHYDROGENASE – Enzyme found especially in the liver, kidneys, striated muscle and the myocardium. Raised levels can be detected in the blood when these organs or tissues are diseased or injured in response to inflammation.

LARYNX – The 'voicebox' in the throat.

LYMPHOCYTES – These are the white cells found in blood normally responsible for fighting disease.

MACROPHAGE – A large white blood cell capable of ingesting foreign bodies (e.g. bacteria) and dead cells.

MAGNETIC RESONANCE IMAGING (MRI) – This is like an X-ray in that pictures of tissues (and in particular, areas of inflammation) can be taken by the MRI machine. Rather than using X-rays, this machine operates uses radio waves to detect the excess water molecules in inflamed tissues.

MAINTENANCE DOSE – A low dose of medicine required to keep an illness from returning or worsening.

MECHANIC'S HANDS – A condition of the hands where the base of the fingernails become thickened, with irregular and distorted cuticles. In addition, the capillary beds become dilated and the finger tips may develop cracked horizontal lines.

MICROCHIMERISM – The presence of a small number of cells which are able to survive after placental transfer from mother to foetus.

MONOCLONAL ANTIBODIES (MAB) – These are 'artificial' antibodies. They have many uses both for diagnostic purposes and in some instances as a mode of treatment. Monoclonal antibodies used as a treatment may for example destroy the blood cells that are causing myositis. A good example of this is Rituximab (Rituxan), which is a monoclonal antibody designed to destroy 'B' lymphocytes which are responsible for the tissue damage in Dermatomyositis and also possibly in Polymyositis.

MONOCYTE – A large white blood cell formed in the bone marrow which enters the blood and migrates into the connective tissue (e.g. muscle) where it matures into a macrophage.

MUSCLE FIBRE – The basic unit of muscle tissue formed by the fusion of groups of individual muscle cells called myocytes.

MYOGLOBIN – Protein only found in muscle tissue, which transports oxygen throughout a muscle fibre.

NUCLEUS – Structure in the centre of each cell which contains the chromosomes with their genetic material.

OEDEMA (EDEMA) – Swelling of soft tissues.

OESOPHAGUS (ESOPHAGUS) – The tube that passes food from the pharynx to the stomach.

PATHOGENESIS – The ability for disease creation.

PATHOLOGY – The study of disease.

PHARYNX – The medical name for the throat i.e. the area between the back of the mouth and the larynx.

PROGNOSIS – Predicted course and outcome of a disorder.

PROXIMAL – Upper part of arms and legs.

RAYNAUD'S DISEASE – A disorder of the blood vessels/capillaries that is marked by recurrent spasm, especially those of the fingers and toes upon exposure to cold. Characterized by pallor, cyanosis (bluish or purplish discoloration) and redness, in succession. Often accompanied by pain.

REFRACTORY – Failing to respond to treatment.

RELAPSE – The re-emergence of disease symptoms.

REMISSION – A state of the disease process when all indications are that the disease has abated. However, remission implies that although under control, the disease may still return at a later date.

RETROSPECTIVE – A type of study that looks back at patients clinical data/information to see if a treatment may have worked.

RHEUMATIC DISEASE – A disease involving the joints and connective tissues (tendons, ligaments, cartilage, bone etc.).

SEROLOGICAL – Blood is composed of red and white blood cells carried throughout the bloodstream in a straw-coloured liquid called serum. Measurement of the many different proteins, antibodies and electrolytes in serum are called serological techniques.

SHAWL SIGN – A flat red rash covering the shoulders and back.

STEROIDS – A group of natural or synthetic compounds, some of which have immunosuppressive activities (e.g. prednisolone/prednisone).

SJOGREN'S SYNDROME – An autoimmune disease affecting the salivary glands giving dry eyes/mouth.

STRICTURE –Narrowing.

SYSTEMIC – Affecting the whole body.

SYSTEMIC LUPUS ERYTHEMATOSUS (LUPUS OR SLE) – An inflammatory connective tissue disease of unknown cause that occurs mainly in women. Characterized in particular by skin rash, fever and arthritis. This is a multi-system disorder, with serious cases involving the kidneys and central nervous system.

TAPER – Reducing the dosage slowly in small amounts.

THYROID – Underactive thyroid function may be the result of an autoimmune condition. Patients diagnosed with one autoimmune disease often have others as well (see Coeliac). Under-active thyroid disease can be treated by thyroxine supplements.

TNFα (Tumour necrosis factor alpha) – A protein that is produced chiefly by monocytes and macrophages that mediates inflammation. Originally observed to induce the destruction of some tumor cells though now shown to also activate of white blood cells (lymphocytes) as part of the immune response.

TYPE 2 MUSCLE FIBRE ATROPHY – A weakness of the muscles caused by long-term steroid treatment.

ULTRASOUND – This is a technique which uses reflected sound waves to see a hidden object (see also MRI). It is now widely used in medicine for example to obtain images of muscle structure, internal organs or the unborn child.

UTI (urinary tract infection) – Patients on immunosuppressive therapies are often more susceptible to common ailments. Urinary tract infections are frequently a complication of such therapies.

VACUOLES – Microscopic 'holes' often seen in cells. Evident in the muscle biopsies of IBM patients.

VASCULITIS – Inflammation of the blood vessels/capillaries.

Acknowledgements

First and foremost, I would like to thank the people with myositis who have been kind enough to update their case studies for this new edition of 'Myositis'. I know that sometimes this can be a painful experience. Thanks also goes to the people who have submitted their case study for the first time. Without all of you this book would not have been possible.

I am indebted to my husband Rob and Dr Bernie Colaço who have helped with the writing and editing of the 'medical' chapters.

I thank all the authors for giving their time voluntarily to write such informative and enlightening chapters. They are: Dr Helene Alexandersson, Dr Geraldine Cambridge, Dr Hector Chinoy, Dr Bernie Colaço, Dr Robert Cooper, Lisa Copen, Theresa Curry, Dr Rob Fenton, Richard Gay, Janet Horton, Audrey Howe, Angela Hunter, Janelle Jones, Julie Mallen, Dr Mona Manghani, Dr John McCarthy, Susan Maillard, Prof William Ollier, Dr Selwyn Richards, Dr Lucy Wedderburn, Dr Fiona Watt, Dr William West, Jo Wilson.

Again, my old workmates from 20+ years ago have done a great job with the typesetting and printing of the book. A big thank you to Angie Wood and Pete Alderman.

Duncan Spilling, thank you for your wonderful new cover design. It's brilliant!

My friends whom I have made since having myositis are such special people. We share an understanding of each other which is unique. You know who you are without me writing your names here. I just want to say how much you all mean to me.

My three children, Nicola, Dani and Charlotte are now independent young women and I am so proud of them. They continue to give me love, support and encouragement. I couldn't have more beautiful daughters! You are all just the best people ever.

I am also grateful to my sister, Roro for her friendship, love and constant encouragement.

There are many more people whom I could mention. Just a few of them are Pam, Annie, Sheila, Bernie and Sarah – thanks for always being there for me.

Lastly, Rob, my husband of 28 years, deserves a very special mention. He has supported me through the writing of my first book and now this, my second book. But most of all he has supported me through what has been a difficult illness to deal with and has never wavered in his kindness and love for me.

Jenny Fenton 2006